T0344927

**Applications of Regression
Models in Epidemiology**

Applications of Regression Models in Epidemiology

Erick Suárez, Cynthia M. Pérez, Roberto Rivera, and Melissa N. Martínez

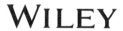

Published by John Wiley & Sons, Inc., Hoboken, New Jersey
Published simultaneously in Canada

For general information on our other products and services or for technical support, please contact our Customer Care Department within the United States at (800) 762-2974, outside the United States at (317) 572-3993 or fax (317) 572-4002.

Wiley also publishes its books in a variety of electronic formats. Some content that appears in print may not be available in electronic formats. For more information about Wiley products, visit our web site at www.wiley.com.

Library of Congress Cataloging-in-Publication Data:

Names: Erick L. Suárez, Erick L., 1953-
Title: Applications of Regression Models in Epidemiology / Erick Suarez [and three others].
Description: Hoboken, New Jersey : John Wiley & Sons, Inc., [2017] | Includes
    index.
Identifiers: LCCN 2016042829| ISBN 9781119212485 (cloth) | ISBN 9781119212508 (epub)
Subjects: LCSH: Medical statistics. | Regression analysis. | Public health.
Classification: LCC RA407 .A67 2017 | DDC 610.2/1–dc23 LC record available at
https://lccn.loc.gov/2016042829

Printed in the United States of America

10 9 8 7 6 5 4 3 2 1

To our loved ones

*To those who have a strong commitment
to social justice, human rights,
and public health.*

Table of Contents

Preface

This book is intended to serve as a guide for statistical modeling in epidemiologic research. Our motivation for writing this book lies in our years of experience teaching biostatistics and epidemiology for different academic and professional programs at the University of Puerto Rico Medical Sciences Campus. This subject matter is usually covered in biostatistics courses at the master's and doctoral levels at schools of public health. The main focus of this book is statistical models and their analytical foundations for data collected from basic epidemiological study designs. This 13-chapter book can serve equally well as a textbook or as a source for consultation. Readers will be exposed to the following topics: linear and multiple regression models, matrix notation in regression models, correlation analysis, strategies for selecting the best model, partial hypothesis testing, weighted least-squares linear regression, generalized linear models, conditional and unconditional logistic regression models, Poisson regression, and programming codes in STATA, SAS, R, and SPSS for different practice exercises. We have started with the assumption that the readers of this book have taken at least a basic course in biostatistics and epidemiology. However, the first chapter describes the basic concepts needed for the rest of the book.

Erick Suárez
University of Puerto Rico, Medical Sciences Campus

Cynthia M. Pérez
University of Puerto Rico, Medical Sciences Campus

Roberto Rivera
University of Puerto Rico, Mayagüez Campus

Melissa N. Martínez
Havas Media International Company

Acknowledgments

We wish to express our gratitude to our departmental colleagues for their continued support in the writing of this book. We are grateful to our colleagues and students for helping us to develop the programming for some of the examples and exercises: Heidi Venegas, Israel Almódovar, Oscar Castrillón, Marievelisse Soto, Linnette Rodríguez, José Rivera, Jorge Albarracín, and Glorimar Meléndez. We would also like to thank Sheila Ward for providing editorial advice. This book has been made possible by financial support received from grant CA096297/CA096300 from the National Cancer Institute and award number 2U54MD007587 from the National Institute on Minority Health and Health Disparities, both parts of the U.S. National Institutes of Health. Finally, we would like to thank our families for encouraging us throughout the development of this book.

About the Authors

Erick Suárez is Professor of Biostatistics at the Department of Biostatistics and Epidemiology of the University of Puerto Rico Graduate School of Public Health. He received a Ph.D. degree in Medical Statistics from the London School of Hygiene and Tropical Medicine. With more than 29 years of experience teaching biostatistics at the graduate level, he has also directed in mentoring and training efforts for public health students at the University of Puerto Rico. His research interests include HIV, HPV, cancer, diabetes, and genetical statistics.

Cynthia M. Pérez is a Professor of Epidemiology at the Department of Biostatistics and Epidemiology of the University of Puerto Rico Graduate School of Public Health. She received an M.S. degree in Statistics and a Ph. D. degree in Epidemiology from Purdue University. Since 1994, she has taught epidemiology and biostatistics. She has directed mentoring and training efforts for public health and medical students at the University of Puerto Rico. Her research interests include diabetes, cardiovascular disease, periodontal disease, viral hepatitis, and HPV infection.

Roberto Rivera is an Associate Professor at the College of Business of the University of Puerto Rico at Mayaguez. He received an M.A. and a Ph.D. degree in Statistics from the University of California in Santa Barbara. He has more than 5 years of experience teaching statistics courses at the undergraduate and graduate levels and his research interests include asthma, periodontal disease, marine sciences, and environmental statistics.

Melissa N. Martínez is a statistical analyst at the Havas Media International Company, located in Miami, FL. She has an MPH in Biostatistics from the University of Puerto Rico, Medical Sciences Campus and currently graduated from the Master of Business Analytics program at National University, San Diego, CA. For the past 7 years, she has been performing statistical analyses in the biomedical research, healthcare, and media advertising fields. She has assisted with the design of clinical trials, performing sample size calculations and writing the clinical trial reports.

1

Basic Concepts for Statistical Modeling

Aim: Upon completing this chapter, the reader should be able to understand the basic concepts for statistical modeling in public health.

1.1 Introduction

It is assumed that the reader has taken introductory classes in biostatistics and epidemiology. Nevertheless, in this chapter we review the basic concepts of probability and statistics and their application to the public health field. The importance of data quality is also addressed and a discussion on causality in the context of epidemiological studies is provided.

Statistics is defined as the science and art of collecting, organizing, presenting, summarizing, and interpreting data. There is strong theoretical evidence backing many of the statistical procedures that will be discussed. However, in practice, statistical methods require decisions on organizing the data, constructing plots, and using rules of thumb that make statistics an art as well as a science.

Biostatistics is the branch of statistics that applies statistical methods to health sciences. The goal is typically to understand and improve the health of a population. A population, sometimes referred to as the target population, can be defined as the group of interest in our analysis. In public health, the population can be composed of healthy individuals or those at risk of disease and death. For example, study populations may include healthy people, breast cancer patients, obese subjects residing in Puerto Rico, persons exposed to high levels of asbestos, or persons with high-risk behaviors. Among the objectives of epidemiological studies are to describe the burden of disease in populations and identify the etiology of diseases, essential information for planning health services. It is convenient to frame our research questions about a population in terms of traits. A measurement made of a population is known as a parameter. Examples are: prevalence of diabetes among Hispanics, incidence of breast

Applications of Regression Models in Epidemiology, First Edition. Erick Suárez, Cynthia M. Pérez, Roberto Rivera, and Melissa N. Martínez.

cancer in older women, and the average hospital stay of acute ischemic stroke patients in Puerto Rico. We cannot always obtain the parameter directly by counting or measuring from the population of interest. It might be too costly, time-consuming, the population may be too large, or unfeasible for other reasons. For example, if a health officer believes that the incidence of hepatitis C has increased in the last 5 years in a region, he or she cannot recommend a new preventive program without any data. Some information has to be collected from a sample of the population, if the resources are limited. Another example is the assessment of the effectiveness of a new breast cancer screening strategy. Since it is not practical to perform this assessment in all women at risk, an alternative is to select at least two samples of women, one that will receive the new screening strategy and another that will receive a different modality.

There are several ways to select samples from a population. We want to make the sample to be as representative of the population as possible to make appropriate inferences about that population. However, there are other aspects to consider such as convenience, cost, time, and availability of resources. The sample allows us to estimate the parameter of interest through what is known as a sample statistic, or statistic for short. Although the statistic estimates the parameter, there are key differences between the statistic and the parameter.

1.2 Parameter Versus Statistic

Let us take a look at the distinction between a parameter and a statistic. The classical concept of a parameter is a numerical value that, for our purposes, at a given period of time is constant, or fixed; for example, the mean birth weight in grams of newborns to Chinese women in 2015. On the other hand, a statistic is a numerical value that is random; for example, the mean birth weight in grams of 1000 newborns selected randomly from the women who delivered in maternity units of hospitals in China in the last 2 years. Coming from a subset of the population, the value of the statistic depends on the subjects that fall in the sample and this is what makes the statistic random. Sometimes, Greek symbols are used to denote parameters, to better distinguish between parameters and statistics. Sample statistics can provide reliable estimates of parameters as long as the population is carefully specified relative to the problem at hand and the sample is representative of that population. That the sample should be representative of the population may sound trivial but it may be easier said than done. In clinical research, participants are often volunteers, a technique known as convenience sampling. The advantage of convenience sampling is that it is less expensive and time-consuming. The disadvantage is that results from volunteers may differ from those who do not volunteer and hence the results may be biased. The process of reaching conclusions about the population based on a sample is known as statistical inference. As long as the data obtained from the sample are representative of the population, we can reach conclusions about the population by using the statistics gathered from the sample, while accounting for the uncertainty around these statistics through probability. Further discussion of sampling techniques in public health can be seen in Korn and Graunbard (1999) and Heeringa et al. (2010).

1.3 Probability Definition

Probability measures how likely it is that a specific event will occur. Simply put, probability is one of the main tools to quantify uncertainty. For any event A, we define $P(A)$ as the probability of A. For any event A, $0 \leq P(A) \leq 1$. When an event has probability of 0.5, it means that it is equally likely that the event will or will not occur. As the probability approaches to 1, an event becomes more likely to occur, and as the probability approaches to 0, the event becomes less likely. Examples of events of interest in public health include exposure to secondhand smoke, diagnosis of type 2 diabetes, or death due to coronary heart disease. Events may be a combination of other events. For example, event "A,B" is the event when A and B occur simultaneously. We define $P(A,B)$ as the probability of "A,B." The probability of two or more events occurring is known as a joint probability; for example, assuming A = HIV positive and B = Female, then $P(A,B)$ indicates the joint probability of a subject being HIV positive and female.

1.4 Conditional Probability

The probability of an event A given that B has occurred is known as a conditional probability and is expressed as $P(A|B)$. That is, we can interpret conditional probability as the probability of A and B occurring simultaneously relative to the probability of B occurring. For example, if we define event B as intravenous drug use and event A as hepatitis C virus (HCV) seropositivity status, then $P(A|B)$ indicates the probability of being HCV seropositive given the subject is an intravenous drug user. Beware: $P(A|B) \neq P(B|A)$. In the expression to the left of the inequality we find how likely A is given that B has occurred, while in the expression to the right of the inequality we find how likely B is given that A has occurred. Another interpretation of $P(A|B)$ can be as follows: given some information (i.e., the occurrence of event B), what is the probability that an event (A) occurs? For example, what is the probability of a person developing lung cancer (A) given that he has been exposed to tobacco smoke carcinogens (B)? Conditional probabilities are regularly used to conduct statistical inference.

Let us assume a woman is pregnant. G is the event that the baby is a girl, and H is the event that the expecting mother is a smoker. Can you guess what $P(G|H)$ is without a calculation? Intuitively, we can guess that it is 0.5, or 50%;

however, in general $P(G)<0.5$, just keep in mind that the male/female ratio at birth varies by countries. That is, the fact that the expecting mother is a smoker has no impact on the chances of giving birth to a girl, $P(G|H) = P(G)$. Two events are independent when the occurrence of one event does not affect the probability of occurrence of the other. When events A and B are independent, then $P(A|B) = P(A)$ and $P(B|A) = P(B)$. Independence implies that $P(A, B) = P(A)P(B)$. For example, the probability that a woman has diabetes (A) and she is a lawyer (B) can be found as the product of the probability that a woman has diabetes times the probability that a woman is a lawyer, if we assume that diabetes diagnosis is independent of professional occupation.

1.5 Concepts of Prevalence and Incidence

In public health there are two important concepts for measuring disease occurrence, prevalence and incidence. The prevalence of a disease is the probability of having the disease at a given point in time; for example, the probability of someone being diagnosed with diabetes in a medical visit. Incidence is the probability that a person with no prior disease will develop disease over some specified time period; for example, the probability of developing lung cancer after 10 years of heavy smoking exposure.

1.6 Random Variables

A random variable, also known as a stochastic variable, has values derived from a function that turns outcomes from the sample space into numbers. Probabilities are assigned to either each value or to ranges of values of the random variable. If the random variable is counting something, then it is a discrete random variable. If the random variable is measuring something (e.g., length, weight, or duration) then it is a continuous random variable. Discrete random variables have integer values. For example, the number of hospitalizations, the number of smokers, or the number of HIV-infected patients. Within any interval, continuous random variables have an infinite amount of possible values. Examples are: the body mass index, blood pressure, or fasting plasma glucose levels of a person.

1.7 Probability Distributions

In epidemiological studies, usually the primary variable in a study, Y, is discrete (an integer number). For example, the number of hospital admissions for chest pain, the number of fractures or sprains seen in an emergency room, the number of incident cancer cases, or the number of people with moderate or severe periodontitis.

Other examples would be the specific result of a clinical evaluation, for example, positive versus negative results from a laboratory test, or presence versus absence of disease. In these cases, the study variable Y is dichotomous, where the variable is coded as follows:

$Y = 1$, to indicate the presence of disease (or testing positive).
$Y = 0$, to indicate the absence of disease (or testing negative).

The specific definition of the random variable Y depends on the epidemiologic study design that is used. In a case–control study, history of exposure is the random variable, where persons with the disease of interest (cases) and persons without the disease of interest (controls) are first selected and then we compare the prevalence of exposure in both groups. In a cohort study, the development of the disease is the random variable, where the exposure and nonexposure groups are first defined and then we compare the incidence of disease in each exposure group. These random variables cannot be determined in advance (their values are defined upon completion of the measurement), but their values or attributes can be determined in probabilistic terms. For example,

- In a case–control study, the habit of smoking in the past cannot be defined until a subject undergoes an interview, but we could determine the probability of this habit based on previous data or under specific assumptions.
- In a cohort study, the development of cervical cancer based on human papilloma virus (HPV) infection status is unknown until the study is completed; however, we could determine the probability of this cancer based on previous data or under specific assumptions.

Therefore, for each value of the random variable Y, we need to identify the corresponding probability:

$$y_1 \;\rightarrow\; p_1$$
$$y_2 \;\rightarrow\; p_2$$
$$\vdots \qquad \vdots$$
$$y_k \;\rightarrow\; p_k$$

where

y_i = ith value of the random variable Y
p_i = probability associated with y_i

Probability distribution functions are used to assign probabilities to values of random variables. Usually, a probability distribution is represented in the Cartesian plane, where the possible values of the random variable are plotted on the X-axis, while the corresponding probabilities are on the Y-axis (see Figure 1.1).

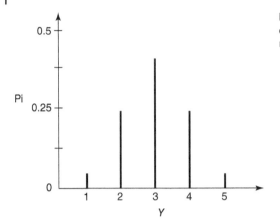

Figure 1.1 Probability distribution of a discrete random variable.

1.8 Centrality and Dispersion Parameters of a Random Variable

The expected value of a random variable is a number that tells us what will be a typical value for the random variable, usually represented as $E(Y)$ or μ. It is not necessarily a possible value of the random variable (a discrete random variable with possible values 1, 2, and 3 might have an expected value of 2.3). In the case of a discrete random variable Y, the expected value of Y is defined as follows:

$$E(Y) = \sum_{i=1}^{n} y_i * p_i \tag{1.1}$$

where p_i indicates the probability of y_i and n is the number of possible values Y can have.

Another characteristic of a random variable is its dispersion, which quantifies how the possible values of Y are spread out around its expected value. Dispersion is usually measured by its variance, $\text{Var}(X)$. It is the mean squared distance from each y_i and the expected value of each possible value of Y. For example, for the discrete random variable Y,

$$\text{Var}(Y) = E[(Y - \mu)^2] = \sum_{i=1}^{n} (y_i - \mu)^2 * p_i \tag{1.2}$$

where μ indicates the expected value of Y and p_i indicates the probability of y_i. Usually, the variance is represented with σ^2. Sometimes the standard deviation, the square root of the variance (σ), is used as a measure of dispersion rather than the variance.

A probability distribution usually depends on one or more parameters that can be estimated with some measurements from a sample selected from the population of interest. For many distributions, a parameter represents the expected value of the measurements, or some function of the expected value. Other parameters may indicate the shape, scale, or width of the distribution (e.g., measures of variability or dispersion). These parameters are important in determining the form of the probability distribution (Jewell, 2004).

1.9 Independence and Dependence of Random Variables

The attribute of independent random variables will be employed frequently in this book. Often, this will be based on the argument that a sample of subjects was chosen randomly. Random selection means that what we obtain as the first observation (first value of a random variable) does not affect the probability of what we will get in the following observation (second value of a random variable). In contrast, when we randomly select households from a sampling design and interview all members of the family of a selected household, it is very likely that their responses will be highly correlated, particularly in dietary habits. For the most part, we will focus on a specific type of dependence between two variables Y, X: linear dependence (e.g., blood pressure (Y) and age (X)). This type of association will be modeled through conditional probabilities (and hence conditional expectations). However, keep in mind that absence of linear dependence does not automatically mean independence in general. The association may be nonlinear but our statistical tools to detect linear dependence may not be able to detect the nonlinear dependence.

1.10 Special Probability Distributions

Previously, the presence or absence of a disease was represented in terms of a random variable, with $Y=1$ indicating presence of the disease and $Y=0$ indicating absence of the disease. There is a wide class of situations that can be represented in terms of such a binary random variable. If we abstractly define $P(Y = 1) = p$, then we can set up a family of probability distributions and use it to define general, simplified ways to find values for characteristics in the population of interest, such as probabilities, $E(Y)$ or Var(Y). We will describe the families of probability distributions most widely used in the statistical analysis of data derived from basic epidemiologic study designs.

1.10.1 Binomial Distribution

A Bernoulli trial is an observation that has two possible outcomes, identified as success or failure (Rosner, 2010). For example, the result of a serological test for HIV represents a Bernoulli trial, since the results of this test can be classified as a random variable with two possible results: positive (success) or negative (failure). The binomial distribution can be used when the random variable represents the number of cases (successes) based on a fixed number of independent Bernoulli trials. The specific formula to obtain probabilities of a binomial random variable is as follows:

$$f(y; n, p) = \frac{n!}{y!(n-y)!} p^y (1-p)^{n-y} \tag{1.3}$$

where

- n is the parameter that defines the number of independent Bernoulli trials.
- p is the parameter that defines the probability of a success for each Bernoulli trial.
- y indicates one of the possible values of the random variable Y, which vary from 0 to n.

It can be shown that for a binomial random variable, $E(Y) = np$, while $Var(Y) = np(1-p)$. For example, assume you want to determine the probability of observing exactly two HIV+ individuals in a hypothetical study where participants were chosen randomly of 20 injection drug users ($n = 20$). If it is known that the probability of being HIV+ is 0.10 ($p = 0.1$), then

$$f(2; 20, 0.1) = \frac{20!}{2!(20-2)!} 0.1^2 (1-0.1)^{20-2} = 0.285$$

That is, there is a 28.5% probability of observing exactly 2 out of 20 HIV+ drug users in this hypothetical study, where the probability of any person being HIV+ is 0.1. Also, in this case $E(Y) = 20(0.1) = 2$. That is, for every sample of 20 injection drug users, we expect two to be HIV+. Moreover, $Var(Y) = 20(0.1)$ $(0.9) = 1.8$. With such a low spread, large values of Y are highly unlikely in this example (readers can double check this by finding probabilities of values of Y close to its largest possible value, 20).

1.10.2 Poisson Distribution

The Poisson distribution can be used when the random variable represents the number of cases (successes) under three conditions:

- i) In a very large number of independent Bernoulli trials when the probability of success is small.
- ii) For a unit of time (e.g., day, month, or year).
- iii) On a unit area (e.g., square meter, square kilometer, or square mile) or volume (e.g., cubic meter or cubic centimeter).

An example of a random variable that could be associated with a Poisson distribution is the number of cancer cases reported in one year in a specific community. Another example would be the number of car accidents that occur in a given week. The formula to find the probability of a specific value of a Poisson random variable is as follows:

$$f(y; \lambda) = \frac{\lambda^y e^{-\lambda}}{y!} \tag{1.4}$$

where

λ is the distribution parameter that indicates the number of cases expected per unit of time or space (area or volume).

y is the value of the random variable. The possible values of a random variable with Poisson distribution range from 0 to infinity ($+\infty$).

e is the Euler constant, whose value is approximately 2.7183.

Furthermore, $E(Y) = \lambda$ and $\text{Var}(y) = \lambda$. For example, assume that in a specific community there is an average of 10 car accidents per week ($\lambda = 10$) and you want to determine the probability of observing 7 car accidents ($Y = 7$). Substituting this parameter in the Poisson formula, we get the following:

$$f(7; 10) = \frac{10^7 e^{-10}}{7!} = 0.09$$

That is, there is a 0.09 probability of observing exactly 7 car accidents in a week in the community, where on average there are 10 car accidents per week.

1.10.3 Normal Distribution

The normal probability distribution is associated with continuous random variables and is used in various situations. One such application arises when it is desired to estimate the average of a random variable through a sample of a population, such as the average weight of newborn infants. Since continuous random variables have infinitive possible values, they demand the definition of a density function; a function with values ≥ 0 for all values of Y and whose area below the function curve totals 1. The *density function* specific to the normal distribution is as follows:

$$f(y; \mu, \sigma^2) = \frac{1}{\sqrt{2\pi\sigma^2}} e^{-((y-\mu)^2)/2\sigma^2} \tag{1.5}$$

where

μ is the parameter that indicates the expected value of the random variable Y.

σ^2 is the parameter defining the variance of Y, that is, the expected value $(y - \mu)^2$.

y indicates the value of the random variable.

e indicates the Euler constant, whose value is approximately 2.7183.

π indicates the constant whose value is approximately 3.1416.

A normally distributed random variable takes values from minus infinity to plus infinity $(-\infty < Y < +\infty)$. The graphical presentation of this density function looks like a bell, that is, a symmetrical distribution such as the one presented in Figure 1.2.

The "top of the bell" is located at $Y = \mu$. For continuous random variables, probabilities for a range of possible values are found as areas under the probability density function, within the range of possible values. In Figure 1.2, as the values of Y deviate from μ, they become less likely to occur, because the associated area under the normal density function becomes smaller. The normal distribution is symmetric around its mean and, therefore, the mean of a normally distributed random variable is equal to its median. For example, to determine the probability that Y is in the range (a, b), you need to get the area under the curve that is generated with this function. That is, calculate the following integral:

$$\int_a^b \frac{1}{\sqrt{2\pi\sigma^2}} e^{-((y-\mu)^2)/2\sigma^2} dy \tag{1.6}$$

For continuous random variables, because the area under the curve at any point is always zero, the probability for a single value of Y *is zero*. However, in discrete probability distributions, such as the binomial distribution and the Poisson distribution, probabilities of exact values of the random variable are not necessarily zero.

The normal distribution will always keep its shape regardless of the values of μ and σ. With this in mind, if Y is normally distributed with mean μ and standard deviation σ, and we define a new random variable

$$Z = \frac{Y - \mu}{\sigma}, \tag{1.7}$$

it can be shown that Z will also follow a normal distribution but with mean 0 and standard deviation 1. Z is known as a standard normal random variable.

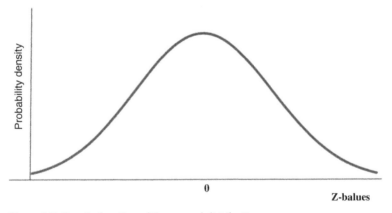

Figure 1.2 Density function of the normal distribution.

The probability for a normally distributed random variable for any μ and σ can be obtained by transforming it to Z.

The normal distribution plays a vital role in the theory of the distribution of the sample mean $\overline{X} = \frac{\sum_{i=1}^{n} x_i}{n}$, assuming X is another continuous random variable. This is in large part due to the central limit theorem, which states the following: Suppose we have a random sample of size n from a population with an arbitrary probability distribution with mean μ and standard deviation σ. The distribution of $\overline{X}$ will tend to a normal distribution as n increases. In fact, the central limit theorem applies even for discrete random variables. These approximated probabilities found through the central limit theorem will allow us to perform inference (e.g., hypothesis testing, confidence intervals, and linear regression) more easily, even when nonnormal random variables are involved (Rosner, 2010). As a rule of thumb, often $n \geq 30$ is sufficient to make the central limit theorem applicable. But care is needed. If you take a careful look at what the central limit theorem says, you will notice that it does not state when the sample size is big enough for $\overline{X}$ to be normally distributed in general. The central limit theorem cannot make such a statement because the adequate sample size will depend on the distribution population, and recall that we may not even know what type of probability distribution the population has. Generally, the more asymmetric the population distribution, the larger the sample size we need for the central limit theorem to hold.

1.11 Hypothesis Testing

One of the objectives of epidemiologic studies is to evaluate a research hypothesis regarding disease etiology. Statistical inference is the process of drawing conclusions based on data, and statistical hypothesis testing is the procedure most used to accomplish that. The principle consists of establishing two mutually exclusive hypotheses: one called the null hypothesis (H_0), the other is referred to as the alternative hypothesis (H_a). For example, newborns have an expected birth weight of 6 lb; however, it is suspected that for smoking mothers the expected birth weight of their child is lower; therefore, assuming a sample of newborn babies of smoking mothers, H_0: $\mu \geq 6$ and H_a: $\mu < 6$.

In hypothesis testing the null hypothesis is assumed to be true, and depending on the data, we decide either to not reject the null hypothesis, or reject it for the alternative. Since there is no way of knowing which of the two hypotheses is correct, we may incur an error when choosing a hypothesis. Two types of error may occur. The null hypothesis may be rejected although it is in fact true—this is known as type I error. We may also not reject the null although it is in fact false—this is known as type II error. The probability of type I error is called the significance level of the test and expressed as α, while the probability of type II error is expressed as β. Both errors are important but we cannot optimize the hypothesis testing procedure by simultaneously reducing the probability of both errors. Instead, in practice an appropriate significance level is chosen, and the hypothesis testing is performed such that we have the highest probability of rejecting the null when it is false (this probability is called the power of the test, or $1 - \beta$). As the sample size increases, the power of the test becomes stronger (hence, β becomes smaller). Typical values of α are 0.05, 0.1, or 0.01. By far, the most common significance level is 0.05. But keep in mind that a significance level should be chosen before looking at the data, and the choice should be based on how serious it would be to incur in type I error in the situation at hand.

The decision to reject or not H_0 depends on the estimate of the parameter of interest. Specifically, the parameter estimate must be far enough from what is stated in the H_0 for the null hypothesis to be rejected. When conducting statistical inference on the population mean μ, the most reliable estimator is the sample mean $\overline{X}$. Returning to the situation when H_0: $\mu \geq 6$ and H_a: $\mu < 6$, then the null hypothesis should be rejected if $\overline{X}$ is too far below 6. The preferred way to measure whether the data contradict the null hypothesis or not is through the p-value: the probability of obtaining a parameter estimate at least as extreme as the observed result when H_0 is true. Hence, if the p-value is low, the observed sample mean is an unusual value under the null hypothesis; this implies that there is not enough evidence to support the null hypothesis H_0 (see Figure 1.3).

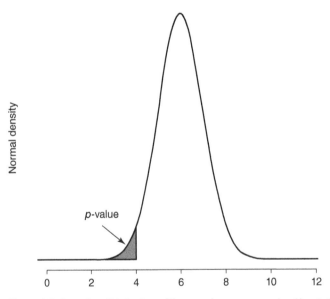

Figure 1.3 Sampling distribution of the sample mean assuming H_0: $\mu \geq 6$. The p-value is based on a sample mean of 4, $Pr[X \leq 4|H_0$ is true], and $n = 100$.

The limit assigned to the p-value is α, because this has been chosen as an acceptable probability of type I error. In summary, if p-value $< \alpha$, we reject H_0; otherwise, we do not. If $\alpha = 0.05$, Rosner (2010) recommends the following guidelines for judging the evidence against the null hypothesis (called significance results):

If $0.01 \leq p$-value <0.05, then the results are significant.
If $0.001 \leq p$-value <0.01, then the results are very significant.
If p-value <0.001, then the results are highly significant.
If p-value >0.05, then the results are considered not statistically significant (sometimes denoted by NS).

However, if $0.05 \leq p$-value <0.1, then a trend toward statistical significance is sometimes noted. Also, it cannot be emphasized enough that α should be chosen as part of the study design before observing the data. As tempting as it may be to rely on guidelines of p-value ranges to determine the strength of the evidence against the null hypothesis, technically the p-value is not a direct measure of evidence against the null hypothesis. The p-value is recording the statistical position of data relative to a hypothesis; it provides an appropriate starting point for inference conclusions (Fraser and Reid, 2016). One of the main problems of using the p-value as a measure of evidence against the null hypothesis is that it is a function of sample size. Specifically, for small n, it becomes more difficult to reject the null hypothesis. On the other hand, if a sample size is large enough, then any arbitrary null hypothesis can be rejected, but caution should be taken to not increase the type II error. For the p-value to be able to directly measure evidence against the null hypothesis, it must measure the probability that H_0 is true. But traditional hypothesis testing methods are not constructed this way.

Among MEDLINE abstracts and PubMed full-text articles with p-values, 96% of them reported at least one p-value ≤ 0.05 (Chavalarias et al., 2016). However, the American Statistical Association has advised researchers to avoid drawing scientific conclusions or making policy decisions purely on the basis of p-values. The validity of scientific conclusions, including their reproducibility, depends on more than the statistical methods themselves. When performing hypothesis testing, it is best to interpret p-values while also taking into account sample size and the *magnitude of the difference between groups* (known as *effect size* or *treatment effect*). Appropriately chosen techniques, properly conducted analyses, and correct interpretation of statistical results also play a key role in ensuring that conclusions are sound and that the uncertainty surrounding them is represented properly (Wasserstein and Lazar, 2016). When assessing hypotheses in epidemiologic studies, the STROBE (*Strengthening the Reporting of Observational Studies in Epidemiology*) guidelines require that all observational studies report unadjusted and confounder-adjusted estimates of the *magnitude of the association (exposure–disease)* along with their confidence intervals. In addition, the guidelines recommend providing information that enables the researchers to test their hypothesis and draw conclusion about the clinical significance of the study findings (Vandenbroucke et al., 2007).

1.12 Confidence Intervals

Rather than estimate an unknown parameter with a (single) number, one can also provide a range of numbers that likely cover the value of the parameter. This is what confidence intervals do. A two-sided confidence interval takes a point estimate of a parameter and subtracts a margin of error to obtain a lower bound for the interval, and adds a margin of error to the point estimate to get an upper bound for the interval. In one-sided confidence intervals, you either subtract or add a margin of error to the point estimate; if you subtract the margin of error, the upper limit is open; if you add the margin of error, the lower limit is open. The margin of error is a function of the standard error of the point estimate and the significance level. The end result is an interval for which there is a prespecified level of confidence that includes the unknown parameter of interest. Typical confidence levels used when constructing confidence intervals are 90, 95, and 99%. For example, if the two-sided 95% confidence interval for the expected birth weight among smoking mothers is between 2.5 and 5.5 lb (95% CI: 2.5, 5.5), this indicates that the expected birth weight could be any value between 2.5 and 5.5 lb with 95% confidence. In other words, for every 100 random samples of smoking mothers, under the same conditions, we are expecting that 95 times the expected value will be within these limits. The appeal of confidence intervals is that they give an idea of the uncertainty in the point estimate. Larger confidence intervals indicate more uncertainty in the point estimate, while smaller confidence intervals indicate less uncertainty.

1.13 Clinical Significance Versus Statistical Significance

When the null hypothesis is rejected, we say that the result is statistically significant. But care is needed when interpreting this in a practical sense. By rejecting the null hypothesis, the data suggest that the set of parameter values stated in H_a is the most likely to be correct. However, the true parameter value may still be so close to the set of values stated in H_0 that from a practical point of view, the results are not important. Many statisticians argue that confidence intervals should be used over hypothesis testing to draw inference since, by providing a measure of uncertainty for the parameter estimate, they are better suited to determine clinical importance. For example, suppose there is a study that aims to determine the effectiveness of a new treatment to reduce levels of low-density lipoprotein cholesterol (LDL-C). The company determines that after 3 months of use, at least a 10 point decrease in LDL-C would be considered clinically important. The study consists of measuring LDL-C of participants before and after 3 months of treatment. If a 95% confidence interval of [−5.2, 2.6] is obtained, then there is neither statistical nor clinical importance. If a 95% confidence interval of [3.4, 11.4] is obtained, then the results are statistically significant, but not clinically important because the lower bound is below 10. If a 95% confidence interval of [12.2, 19.7] is obtained, then the results are both statistically significant and practically important.

1.14   Data Management

Data management is a topic that is often omitted in statistics courses. However, when performing statistical inference, proper data management is of foremost importance. The aim of data management is to access the data as quickly as possible while ensuring the best quality of the data. For projects requiring thousands of measurements on subjects, error is virtually guaranteed to occur. Poor quality data will not represent the population of interest well and hence lead to misleading statistical inference. Effective data management minimizes data errors and missing values, resulting in less reanalysis of the data. This can translate into adequate statistical inference, and savings in time, resources, and costs. Although some entities provide guidelines on data management, in this section we summarize the components of data management to help ensure the proper management and high quality of data.

For data management, it is best to establish a protocol to ensure data quality. A data quality protocol can be established for each of the following stages of research before data analysis (Pandav et al., 2002):

- study design
- data collection/measurement
- data entry/recording
- data processing
- screening the data

Each stage affects data quality. A data quality protocol establishes a coherent data management procedure that ensures efficient creation and use of research data. We address below the most important aspects of each stage of research.

1.14.1   Study Design

Through the study design, the researcher intends to answer questions of interest as effectively as possible. When it comes to data management, the steps taken at this stage of the research have an impact on quality of data (Richesson and Andrews, 2012).

- *Specification of hypotheses and design of testing mechanisms.* Hypotheses are stated according to the questions of interest. Careful consideration is needed to obtain the right data and to use the right analysis to obtain answers to the questions of interest.
- *Choice of study instruments.* The study instrument chosen affects the precision of observations through the type of technology, and ease of instrument use for both staff and study participants. Standardization of data collection procedures is key to maximizing the uniformity of the data obtained. Study rehearsal in a fashion similar to the actual study is crucial to pretest instruments and detect flaws. For example, pretesting of a study questionnaire, also known as a pilot run, assesses clarity of questions, appropriateness of chosen categories, presence of sensitive questions, and general flow of questions.
- *Creating a manual of procedures.* The manual provides easily accessible information on data quality protocols to all staff involved. For example, detailed instructions for interviews are provided.
- *Staff training.* Guidelines for staff training are presented to and discussed with personnel according to their role in carrying out the study (e.g., effective and standard use of instruments, protocols to use in case of problems, and how to process data effectively.)
- *Updates in study procedures.* Changes are inevitable in a study. Research team members must be notified of pertinent changes to maintain study continuity and avoid problems. Some changes occur almost automatically, but others require decisions from key personnel. For example, some diseases do not have gold standards for diagnosis. Major changes in the diagnosis criteria may occur based on independent work while the study is ongoing. The key personnel will determine the potential impact of these changes and alternative ways to address them (e.g., perhaps by diagnosing the disease by the traditional criteria and also the new criteria, assuming resources allow this).

It must be recognized that just because the study design was done well, it does not mean that there will not be errors or that data will be of high quality. The study must be monitored to ensure the implementation proceeds as designed. Furthermore, efficient data collection and data entry are also key.

1.14.2 Data Collection

The task of measuring and gathering information on processes of interest is known as data collection. This information is typically represented in terms of variables. One must ensure data redundancy and consistency of the data collection procedures. Data may be primary or secondary. Primary data are collected firsthand by the research team, while secondary data come from another source and perhaps were intended for a purpose other than that of the study of interest.

1.14.3 Data Entry

The analysis of the data requires its entry into a computer in digital form. Sometimes, data collection and data entry occur simultaneously, but this is not always the case. Some recommendations on how to do data entry efficiently are described below:

- Use code when possible. For example, if age will be recorded multiple times, enter date of birth and date of measurement to determine age. Often measurements on several subjects are performed in a day. Therefore, fewer individual entries are needed when entering date of measurement instead of actual age. As a result, human error is reduced.
- Use appropriate software for data entry. User-friendly software with the ability to recognize and minimize errors is recommended.
- Keep a record of codification, also known as a dictionary or codebook. A dictionary prevents relying on memory when returning to the data and hence leads to fewer errors. It also makes it easier to share the data for different kinds of analysis, and helps in building convenient, consistent codification based on similar variables for future measurements. The dictionary should include the following:
  - Variable abbreviation used.
  - Definition of variable (continuous or discrete?).
  - If a variable is numerical, unit of measurement must be specified.
  - Definition of coded values for categorical variables (e.g., M = male, F = female, or 1 = female, 0 = male).
  - An explanation of how levels of categorical variables are defined when coming from numerical measurements.
  - Use intuitive names for variables. For example, use gender for gender abbreviation instead of X4 so that it is easily recognized. Keep variable names consistent through follow-up. The more variables one has, the more important it is to make variable names recognizable and consistent.
  - Limit use of codification of categories of variables. For example, writing 1 for male and 0 for female is convenient for analysis but not necessarily for data entry, and it is best avoided. If one chooses to use codification (say because codification is already present for past measurements of a variable), keep codification of qualitative variables consistent. For example, if smoking status at baseline is defined as 0 for nonsmoker, 1 for exsmoker, and 2 for current smoker, future measurements should use the same coding. Refer to the dictionary of variables if necessary to ensure consistent codification.

When sharing data involving human subjects, one must remember to protect the privacy and confidentiality and only share the necessary part of the data, excluding information that identifies participants. Also, define missing values appropriately and be careful in treating missing values as a category for categorical data.

1.14.4 Data Screening

Probably the most underappreciated step of data management is data screening. It consists of checking data for unusual observations. It is a procedure conducted before analysis, during exploratory analysis, and when conducting diagnostics on the inferential methods to be used. Unusual observations may be correct, but may also be due to errors or due to sampling issues (e.g., questions or answers were not understood by study respondents). Sometimes data issues are straightforward to detect. For example, one may find that a participant's height was entered as 150 in., and the issue would potentially be detected when diagnostics of the models are made. But data issues are not always easy to detect. A height may be erroneously entered as 65 in. and hence, go undetected on its own. But if the data are screened in conjunction with the person's age, we could detect the error, especially if the person is too young to have such height (e.g., the person is 2-years old). For categorical variables, issues likely would not be detected when diagnostics of the model are made. In what follows, we provide some tips for data screening:

- Start screening data early in the project. By starting early one can change patterns of ineffective data entry, data collection, or correct errors by contacting respondents.
- Screen data regularly. This includes data audits, where data management staff checks if the participant's identification number in the data set can be traced back to original documents and other tasks. Missing values or skipping patterns by study subjects may indicate privacy concerns, or other type of issues that demand attention. Any flaws or concerns should be properly documented.
- Check if observations are feasible. For example, are there values of weight or height that are simply impossible? This can be done through numerical and graphical summaries to detect 'abnormalities.' Maximum and minimum values are very useful for quantitative variables.
- Calculate error rates over all variables and per variable. Büchele et al. (2005) suggest ways to determine error rates.
- Counts should be made of nonchanging categorical variables at different time points. For example, one can check if the total number of males and females at baseline matches with the total number of males and females at follow-up.

One must be aware that, although mismatching counts indicate an issue (assuming no missing values in gender), matching counts do not necessarily mean there is no issue, since multiple input errors may cancel each other out.

- Similar to the preceding tip, one can check numerical data with *a priori* predictable changes to detect issues. For example, if baseline and follow-up measurements are approximately 2 years apart, age of subject should range between 1 and 3 years.
- Refer to original data collection forms when in doubt.
- Do categorical entries at different time points make sense? For example, if a person at baseline says he formerly smoked, at follow-up, an entry of never smoked is a sign that something is wrong.
- Plot the data (dot plots, histograms, and scatter plots). Plots help us explore features of the population of interest but also help us detect data issues. For example, suppose data include two quantitative variables: an age variable and a years-of-education variable. You should not expect a 15-year-old individual to have over 20 years of education. A scatterplot would be able to detect this type of issue.
- Search rows of observations for unlikely combination of variable values. This method allows screening of categorical and quantitative data. Returning to the age and education example, suppose education is categorical (less than high school, high school, bachelor's degree, master's degree, and doctoral degree), it is unlikely that a 10-year-old individual would have a doctoral degree. As another example, a male subject cannot be pregnant. A search will easily detect these types of data issues.
- If multiple people are in charge of data entry, ensure use of dictionary and communication between personnel.
- While conducting exploratory analysis, screening the data through plots and diagnostics is advised. Note that data errors are different than errors in analysis. Diagnostics help us detect both!
- During analysis, be sure to back up data and the analysis code. It is also helpful to include comments in analysis code for future reference.

1.14.5 What to Do When Detecting a Data Issue

- Try to determine if there is an error from original data or from primary source, including contacting personnel who collected/recorded data or the study subjects. Contact personnel within and outside the data management branch for necessary adjustments.
- If the issue is resolved, make a record of the data issue, so that others using the data for analysis are aware. Also, if source of error can be avoided, bring up the error source to the appropriate research team to avoid further errors.

- If the issue is not resolved, record the issue in a log. The data may be turned into a missing value during analysis depending on the extent of the error. There are several ways to deal with missing values. It is not uncommon with categorical variables to define a category of missing and use it for analysis. However, this action is not recommended due to unpredictable bias that likely results from this method (see Chapter 25 in Gelman and Hill, 2007).

1.14.6 Impact of Data Issues and How to Proceed

It is important to distinguish between data issues, data quality, and information quality. Data issues are mishaps with the data. Many of the issues detected in the data will have no impact on the analysis. Whether a data issue deserves attention is dependent on the severity of the issue and the aim of the analysis. If the information quality of your data is poor, then the data are useless.

There are many definitions of data quality. We prefer to define it as a measure of data issues. The more data issues detected, the poorer the quality of data. This definition is adequate in the sense that it may still be appropriate to rely on medium or poor quality data to perform statistical inference. This will depend on the aim of the statistical procedure.

It is not always possible to implement a protocol to limit the number of data issues, and even when this is done, data issues may still occur. Furthermore, data may already be available to perform statistical inference and the data may have issues. Two things must be considered in these situations. First, data should be screened to have an indication of the quality of the data. Remember that this is a function of the number of issues and the aims of a study. Second, if data quality is a concern, then there are statistical procedures that help diminish the impact of data issues. Data quality problems can affect the performance of traditional statistical models. For example, in situations when data errors lead to many values that are very far from the mean (i.e., many outliers), the assumption of a normal distribution becomes inadequate. An alternative is the use of robust estimators, which help minimize the effect of misspecifying the model.

When studying the association among variables, an option is measurement error models, also known as regression with errors in variables. Chapter 2 reviews simple linear regression, a method that assumes that the response variable Y is measured with error but that the explanatory variable X is measured without error. Considerable error in X will lead to biased estimates of slope coefficients and hence potentially to wrong conclusions about the association between Y and X. This idea obviously applies as well when performing other types of regression. Measurement error models account for the fact that explanatory variables are measured with error. When in doubt of the quality of the data, a conservative move is to apply both traditional regression models and measurement error models to see if there are major differences in the results. For the rest of this book, we work with either data of good quality, or data that have already been screened and processed for quality unless otherwise stated.

1.15   Concept of Causality

One of the central objectives of epidemiology is to assess the causal role of specific exposures in the occurrence of disease or other health outcomes of interest. In addition to making predictions about disease risk, regression models are also used in epidemiology to assess the causal role of selected exposures while controlling for confounding variables. Although the concept of causality is complex, several guidelines have been proposed to assess whether there is a causal relationship between an exposure and health outcome (Rothman et al., 2012). Although a detailed discussion of the framework that has been developed to judge causation is beyond the scope of this book, we outline the guidelines proposed by Sir Austin Bradford Hill in 1965 (Hill, 1965; Fraser and Reid, 2015).

- **Strength of Association:** Strength measures the magnitude of the association between exposure and disease. The greater the strength of association, the greater the evidence that the association is one of cause and effect.
- **Biological Gradient:** The biological gradient, or dose–response evidence, suggests that the higher the level, intensity, or duration of exposure, the greater the risk of developing the disease under study.
- **Temporal Sequence:** The timing assumes that the exposure factor precedes the development of the disease under study.
- **Consistency of Findings:** Consistency means that the observed association between exposure and disease is similar to previous studies with different designs and different populations. That is, the study findings may be reproducible.
- **Biological Plausibility of the Hypothesis:** Biological plausibility means that the observed association is compatible with the existing knowledge about the pathophysiology of the disease. However, the absence of this criterion is not sufficient to exclude causality as the current knowledge may be inadequate to explain the observed association.
- **Coherence:** This criterion implies that the study findings do not conflict with existing theory and current knowledge. This approach combines aspects of biological compatibility and biological plausibility.
- **Specificity of the Association:** The specificity indicates that the factor or cause under study produces the disease and that the disease must result from a single cause.

- **Experimental Evidence:** The experiment requires studies of different nature (clinical trials, community trials, and laboratory studies) in order to provide evidence for causation.
- **Analogy:** If a similar agent exerts similar effects, then it is more likely that the association is causal.

With the exception of a temporal sequence, the other criteria mentioned above cannot be considered as both necessary and sufficient to prove causality. Due to the inherent limitations of these criteria, some recommend a refutationism approach, in which repeated observations do not lead to the formulation of a natural law, but only the belief that such a law has been found (Rothman et al., 2012).

Prior to deriving causal inferences in epidemiologic studies, the internal and external validity of the study findings must be thoroughly assessed. Internal validity implies that the study results and conclusions are valid for the study group. Thus, this type of validity requires that there are no other plausible explanations (e.g., sources of potential bias, confounding, and chance) for the observed findings. External validity refers to the extent to which the results from a study can be generalized to a target population from which the sample was retrieved. An understanding of the potential threats to study validity is essential in order to derive valid inferences from the findings generated in epidemiologic studies.

References

Büchele, G., Och, B., Bolte, G., and Weiland S.K. (2005) Single vs. double data entry. *Epidemiology*, **16**, 130–131.

Chavalarias, D., Wallach, J.D., Li, A.H., and Ioannidis, J.P. (2016) Evolution of reporting p values in the biomedical literature, 1990–2015. *JAMA*, **315**, 1141–1148.

Fraser, D. and Reid, N. (2016) *Crisis in science? Or crisis in statistics! Mixed messages in statistics with impact on science.* Journal of Statistics Research, **1**, 48–50.

Heeringa, S.G., West, B.T., and Berglund, P.A. (2010) *Applied Survey Data Analysis.* Boca Raton, FL: Chapman & Hall/CRC.

Hill, A.B. (1965) The environment and disease: association or causation? *Proc. R Soc, Med.*, **58**, 295–300.

Gelman, A. and Hill, J. (2007) *Data Analysis Using Regression and Multilevel/ Hierarchical Models.* New York, NY: Cambridge University Press.

Jewell, N. (2004) *Statistics for Epidemiology,* Boca Raton, FL: Chapman & Hall/ CRC.

Korn, E.L. and Graunbard, B.I. (1999) *Analysis of Health Surveys*, John Wiley & Sons, Inc.

Pandav, R., Mehta, A., Belle, S.H., Martin, D.E., Chandra, V., Dodge, H.H., and Ganguli, M. (2002) Data management and quality assurance for an international project: The Indo–US Cross-National Dementia Epidemiology Study. *Int. J. Geriatr. Psychiatry*, **17**, 510–518.

Richesson, R.L. and Andrews, J.E. (eds) (2012) *Clinical Research Informatics*. London, UK: Springer.

Rosner, B. (2010) *Fundamentals of Biostatistics*, 7th edition. Boston, MA: Cengage Learning.

Rothman, K.J., Greenland, S., and Lash, T.L. (2012) *Modern Epidemiology*, 3rd edition. Philadelphia, PA: Lippincott Williams & Wilkins.

Vandenbroucke, J.P., von Elm, E., Altman, D.G., Gøtzsche, P.C., Mulrow, C.D., Pocock, S.J., Poole, C., Schlesselman, J.J., and Egger, M. (2007) STROBE Initiative. Strengthening the Reporting of Observational Studies in Epidemiology (STROBE): explanation and elaboration. *Epidemiology*, **18**, 805–835.

Wasserstein, R.L. and Lazar, N.A. (2016) The ASA's statement on *p*-values: context, process, and purpose. *Am. Stat.*, **70**:(2), 129–133.

2

Introduction to Simple Linear Regression Models

Aim: Upon completing this chapter, the reader should be able to apply simple linear regression models to evaluate relationships between a quantitative random variable and a quantitative variable in public health problems.

2.1 Introduction

Regression models in public health have been used to evaluate a relationship between different variables or characteristics of interest in the community. One purpose of these models is to provide evidence of a possible cause–effect relationship in an epidemiologic study (see section 1.15). This chapter describes the case of simple linear regression model, which allows us to establish a linear relationship between two quantitative variables. In the simple regression model, one of the variables is identified as the *response* or *dependent* variable, while the second is called the *predictor*, *explanatory*, or *independent* variable. Examples of such relationships include the infant's birth weight (response variable) according to maternal age (predictor variable), blood pressure levels by age, cholesterol levels according to the amount of dietary fat intake, and the level of body mass index (BMI) per average weekly consumption of sugar-sweetened beverages. The statistical procedures to evaluate this type of association are summarized in this chapter. Throughout the chapter, the *dependent* variable or *response* will be identified with the letter Y, while for the *independent* or *predictor* variable the letter X will be used. The variable X is regularly associated with the cause or precipitating factor of a condition of interest. In an epidemiological study, the variable Y will be the outcome related to a clinical condition of interest and X is associated with the exposure to the possible cause of this disease (Gordis, 2014).

Applications of Regression Models in Epidemiology, First Edition. Erick Suárez, Cynthia M. Pérez, Roberto Rivera, and Melissa N. Martínez.
© 2017 John Wiley & Sons, Inc. Published 2017 by John Wiley & Sons, Inc.

2.2 Specific Objectives

The specific aims of this chapter are to

- Introduce the concept of simple linear regression.
- Identify the components and basic assumptions of the simple linear regression model.
- Use least-squares method for parameter estimation in a simple linear regression model.
- Evaluate a statistical hypothesis regarding the parameters of the simple linear regression model.
- Estimate the percentage of variation of the dependent variable explained by the simple linear regression model.
- Estimate the expected value through a simple linear regression model.
- Evaluate the behavior of the residuals in a simple linear regression model.
- Interpret the results of a simple linear regression model generated by the statistical software STATA.
- Apply a simple linear regression model to study a problem in public health.

2.3 Model Definition

The value of a quantitative random variable can be expressed as its expected value (μ_Y) plus a random term for each subject, as follows:

$$Y_i = \mu_Y + e_i \tag{2.1}$$

where μ_Y is a constant and e_i is a random error with zero mean and common σ^2 for all observations. The subscript i indicates the particular subject, $i = 1, 2, \ldots, n$.

Suppose there is a quantitative variable X that can be informative of Y, then we can use it to explain the expected value of Y $(\mu_{Y|X})$. In the simplest relationship, we can use the equation of the line as follows:

$$\mu_{Y|X} = \beta_0 + \beta_1 \times X \tag{2.2}$$

where

Y indicates the dependent or response variable.

X indicates the predictor variable (independent variable) and is assumed to be measured without error.

β_1 indicates the parameter (constant) associated with the predictor variable X. It is known as the slope of the regression line, which indicates the change in the expected value of Y per unit change in X.

β_0 indicates the expected value of Y when $X = 0$. It is known as the intercept of the regression line.

If $\beta_1 > 0$, then an increase in X is associated with an increase in $\mu_{Y|X}$. If $\beta_1 < 0$, then an increase in X is associated with a decrease in $\mu_{Y|X}$. If $\beta_1 = 0$, then the variable X does not contribute linearly to the explanation of the expected value of Y. The intercept, β_0, can be interpreted only in special occasions where it is possible that $X = 0$. For example, if the predictor is centered, each value of X is subtracted by its mean $(X - \overline{X})$, then $\mu_{Y|X} = \beta_0 + \beta_1 * (X - \overline{X})$; as a consequence, $\mu_{Y|X} = \beta_0$ when $X = \overline{X}$. However, for mathematical convenience, the intercept usually is kept in the model even when there is no direct interest in its interpretation.

Therefore, a simple linear regression model (SLRM) is regularly defined for specific X values through the following expression:

$$y_i = \beta_0 + \beta_1 x_i + e_i \tag{2.3}$$

where

y_i indicates the specific value of Y for the ith subject.
e_i indicates a random error for the ith subject.
x_i indicates the specific value of X for the ith subject.

If we know the values of the coefficients β_0 and β_1, we can predict the expected value of Y for a subject or group of subjects with a specific value of X. For example, assuming $\beta_0 = 4$ and $\beta_1 = 3$, the value of $\mu_{Y|X}$ for different values of X will be as follows:

Subject	x_i	$\mu_{y_i|x_i} = 4 + 3x_i$
1	5	19
2	6	22
3	10	34

An example would be the relationship between weight and height represented by the following expression:

$$\mu_{weight_i|height_i} = \beta_0 + \beta_1 height_i$$

where

$weight_i$ indicates the response or dependent variable in the ith subject.
$\mu_{weight_i|height_i}$ indicates the expected value of weight in the ith subject, which is explained by the variable *height* using the SLRM.
$height_i$ indicates the value of the variable height in the ith subject. This is the predictor or independent variable in the SLRM.

Another representation of the SLRM is

$$\text{weight}_i = \beta_0 + \beta_1 \text{height}_i + e_i$$

where

e_i indicates a random error for the ith subject under the SLRM.

In general, statistical models are those where the response variable can be expressed as the sum of the following components:

$$\text{response variable} = \text{systematic component} + \text{error component}$$

The systematic component describes the variation of Y that could be explained by specific values of X under the model ($\beta_0 + \beta_1 \text{height}_i$). The remaining variation of Y is defined as the *error component* (e_i), and corresponds to the variation in Y that cannot be explained by the predictor. This term accounts for measurement error, other predictors that either were not included in the model or were not measured, and other sources of uncertainty in the model. In a simple regression model, e_i recognizes the fact that X is not likely to account fully for the variation in Y.

2.4 Model Assumptions

The classical procedure for hypothesis testing on the coefficients of a SLRM is performed under the following assumptions:

i) An equation of a *straight line* exists that determines the functional relationship between the expected value Y and X, as follows:

$$\mu_{Y|X} = \beta_0 + \beta_1 X$$

ii) The error terms are independent.
iii) For the purpose of making significance tests, the error terms are normally distributed:

$$e_i \sim \text{NID}\left(0, \sigma^2\right)$$

where NID stands for "normally and independently distributed" with expected value zero and σ^2 is the common variance for all subjects. This assumption implies that Y_i is normally distributed with mean $\beta_0 + \beta_1 X_i$ and a common variance σ^2.

It should be noted that for our purposes, models are linear on the coefficients. Thus, $\log(Y_i) = \beta_0 + \beta_1 x_i + e_i$ is considered a linear model as is $Y_i = \beta_0 + \beta_1 \sin(x_i) + e_i$. On the other hand, $Y_i = \beta_0 + e^{\beta_1 x_i}$ is not considered linear on the slope. As long as the model is linear in the parameters, the estimation of the coefficients proceeds the same as described in section 2.7.

Figure 2.1 Example of scatterplot.

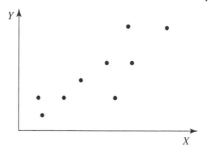

2.5 Graphic Representation

The first step in establishing a possible linear relationship between two variables is through constructing a scatterplot (Figure 2.1). Dots in Figure 2.1 indicate coordinates (x_i, y_i) that are related to the values of the response variable (Y) and the predictor variable (X) for each subject. If there is an imaginary line with slope not equal to zero that can explain the relationship between variables X and Y, then we can assume that a SLRM may explain the increase or decrease of the variable Y. If the trend is increasing, in other words, for an increase in X an increase in Y is observed, the slope of the line should be positive. If the trend is decreasing, that is, for an increase in X a decrease in Y is observed, the slope of the line should be negative. If there is no indication of a linear trend in the changes of Y for changes in X, then it is not possible to justify a linear association between variables Y and X.

2.6 Geometry of the Simple Regression Model

The trend line of the association between X and Y through the linear regression model can be displayed as a linear equation, in the simplest relationship (Figure 2.2).

Figure 2.2 Linear regression model.

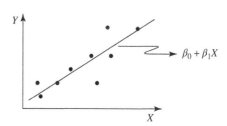

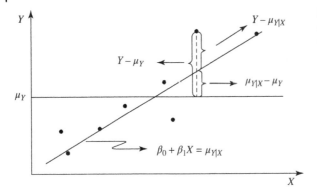

Figure 2.3 Geometry of a simple linear regression model.

The identification of each error (e_i) allows us to evaluate the distance between Y and its expected value under the model $\left(Y_i - \mu_{Y|X}\right)$, which can be expressed as follows:

$$\left(Y_i - \mu_{Y|X}\right) = \left(Y_i - \mu_Y\right) - \left(\mu_{Y|X} - \mu_Y\right)$$

These differences are represented in Figure 2.3.

2.7 Estimation of Parameters

The least-squares method is one of the procedures used to estimate the model parameters β_0 and β_1 from the model $Y_i = \beta_0 + \beta_1 X + e_i$. This procedure determines the values of β_0 and β_1 that minimize the sum of squared errors e_i, and is based on the following expression:

$$S(\beta_0, \beta_1) = \sum e_i^2 = \sum (Y_i - \beta_0 - \beta_1 x_i)^2 \tag{2.4}$$

The values that minimize the function S are identified as *point estimators* of β_0 and β_1, which are represented by $\hat{\beta}_0$ and $\hat{\beta}_1$. These estimators are obtained through differential calculus techniques (Draper and Smith, 1998; Bingham and Fry, 2010). The steps to obtain these estimates are as follows:

i) Taking the partial derivatives of S with respect to each parameter:

$$\frac{\partial S}{\partial \beta_1} = -2 \sum_{i=1}^{n} x_i \left(y_i - \beta_0 - \beta_1 x_i\right) \tag{2.5}$$

$$\frac{\partial S}{\partial \beta_0} = -2 \sum_{i=1}^{n} \left(y_i - \beta_0 - \beta_1 x_i\right) \tag{2.6}$$

ii) Set the derivatives equal to zero:

$$\sum_{i=1}^{n} x_i (y_i - \beta_0 - \beta_1 x_i) = 0 \tag{2.7}$$

$$\sum_{i=1}^{n} (y_i - \beta_0 - \beta_1 x_i) = 0 \tag{2.8}$$

iii) Simplify the two equations (known as *model normal equations*):

$$\hat{\beta}_0 \sum_{i=1}^{n} x_i + \hat{\beta}_1 \sum_{i=1}^{n} x_i^2 = \sum_{i=1}^{n} x_i y_i \tag{2.9}$$

$$\hat{\beta}_0 n + \hat{\beta}_1 \sum_{i=1}^{n} x_i = \sum_{i=1}^{n} y_i \tag{2.10}$$

iv) Obtain the solutions for $\hat{\beta}_1$ and $\hat{\beta}_0$:

$$\hat{\beta}_1 = \frac{\sum_{i=1}^{n} (x_i - \bar{x})(y_i - \bar{y})}{\sum_{i=1}^{n} (x_i - \bar{x})^2} = \frac{\sum_{i=1}^{n} (x_i - \bar{x}) y_i}{\sum_{i=1}^{n} (x_i - \bar{x})^2} \tag{2.11}$$

$$\hat{\beta}_0 = \bar{y} - \hat{\beta}_1 \bar{x} \tag{2.12}$$

2.8 Variance of Estimators

The variances of the regression coefficients' estimators are deducted as follows:

$$\text{var}(\hat{\beta}_1) = \text{var}\left(\frac{\sum_{i=1}^{n}(x_i - \bar{x})(y_i - \bar{y})}{\sum_{i=1}^{n}(x_i - \bar{x})^2}\right) = \left(\frac{\sum_{i=1}^{n}(x_i - \bar{x})^2 \text{var}(y_i)}{\left(\sum_{i=1}^{n}(x_i - \bar{x})^2\right)^2}\right)$$

$$= \frac{\sigma^2 \sum_{i=1}^{n}(x_i - \bar{x})^2}{\left(\sum_{i=1}^{n}(x_i - \bar{x})^2\right)^2} = \frac{\sigma^2}{\sum_{i=1}^{n}(x_i - \bar{x})^2} \tag{2.13}$$

$$\text{var}(\hat{\beta}_0) = \text{var}(\bar{y} - \hat{\beta}_1 \bar{x}) = \text{var}(\bar{y}) + \bar{x}^2 \, \text{var}(\hat{\beta}_1) = \sigma^2 \left(\frac{1}{n} + \frac{\bar{x}^2}{\sum_{i=1}^{n}(x_i - \bar{x})^2}\right) \tag{2.14}$$

where (2.13) uses $\sum_{i=1}^{n} (x_i - \bar{x})(y_i - \bar{y}) = \sum_{i=1}^{n} (x_i - \bar{x}) y_i$ and (2.14) relies on independence of $\bar{y}$ and $\hat{\beta}_1$. The square root of the variances of these estimates is called the standard error of $\hat{\beta}_0$ and $\hat{\beta}_1$:

$$\text{se}(\hat{\beta}_0) = \sqrt{\text{var}(\hat{\beta}_0)}$$

$$\text{se}(\hat{\beta}_1) = \sqrt{\text{var}(\hat{\beta}_1)}$$

The estimate of the variance of Y under the model is

$$\widehat{\mathrm{Var}}\left(Y|X\right) = \hat{\sigma}_{Y|X}^2 = s_{Y|X}^2 = \frac{\sum_{i=1}^{n}\left(y_i - \hat{y}_i\right)^2}{n-2} \tag{2.15}$$

where $\hat{y}_i = \hat{\beta}_0 + \hat{\beta}_1^* x_i$.

2.9 Hypothesis Testing About the Slope of the Regression Line

To evaluate evidence for a linear association between the dependent variable and the independent variable, one must assess whether the slope parameter β_1 in the linear model is different from zero. That is, the hypothesis $H_0 : \beta_1 = 0$ versus $H_a : \beta_1 \neq 0$ must be evaluated. For this evaluation, we have two alternatives: using the Student's t-distribution or using the Fisher's F-distribution through an analysis of variance (ANOVA).

2.9.1 Using the Student's *t*-Distribution

To evaluate H_0, we need to calculate the following statistic:

$$\hat{t} = \frac{\hat{\beta}_1}{\sqrt{\widehat{\mathrm{Var}}\left(\hat{\beta}_1\right)}} \tag{2.16}$$

where

$$\widehat{\mathrm{Var}}(\hat{\beta}_1) = \frac{\hat{\sigma}_{y|x}^2}{\sum_{i=1}^{n}\left(X_i - \overline{X}\right)^2}$$

Under the null hypothesis, $\hat{t}$ follows a t-distribution with $n-2$ degrees of freedom. The assessment of the t-statistic (2.16) can be done by the critical value method, computing the p-value, or through the construction of a confidence interval (Draper and Smith, 1998; Bingham and Fry, 2010).

2.9.2 Using ANOVA

Another alternative to evaluate H_0 is to decompose the numerator of the variance of Y into two independent components named *sources of variation* as follows:

$$\sum_{i=1}^{n}\left(y_i - \overline{y}\right)^2 = \sum_{i=1}^{n}\left(y_i - \hat{y}_i\right)^2 + \sum_{i=1}^{n}\left(\hat{y}_i - \overline{y}\right)^2 \tag{2.17}$$

where

$$\hat{y}_i = \hat{\beta}_0 + \hat{\beta}_1 x$$
denotes the estimate of the value of Y for observation i under the model.

$$SST = \sum_{i=1}^{n} (y_i - \bar{y})^2$$
denotes the total sum of squares, which represents the total variation of Y around its mean ($\bar{y}$).

$$SSE = \sum_{i=1}^{n} (y_i - \hat{y}_i)^2$$
denotes the sum of squared errors, which represents the variation of Y around its fitted value ($\hat{y}_i$).

$$SSR = \sum_{i=1}^{n} (\hat{y}_i - \bar{y})^2$$
denotes the sum of squares due to the regression, which represents the variation of the fitted values of Y ($\hat{y}_i$) around the mean value of Y ($\bar{y}$).

The ratio of the sum of squares to their degrees of freedom is called *mean squares*, which are expressed as follows:

$MSR = SSR/1$ denotes the mean squares due to the regression and
$MSE = SSE/(n - 2)$ denotes the mean squares due to the errors.

The expected values of MSR and MSE are obtained by the following expressions:

$$E(MSR) = \sigma^2 + \beta_1^2 \sum_{i=1}^{n} (x_i - \bar{x})^2 \tag{2.18}$$

$$E(MSE) = \sigma^2 \tag{2.19}$$

Therefore, when $H_0: \beta_1 = 0$ is true,

$$\frac{E(MSR)}{E(MSE)} = \frac{\sigma^2 + \beta_1^2 \sum_{i=1}^{n} (x_i - \bar{x})^2}{\sigma^2} = 1$$

If the variation attributed to the regression model is greater than the variation attributed to the errors, both adjusted by their degrees of freedom, as described in Table 2.1, then this is considered evidence against H_0.

Table 2.1 ANOVA for a simple linear regression model.

Source of variation	Degrees of freedom	Sum of squares	Mean squares	Statistic F_{cal}
Regression (Explained variation)	1	SSR	MSR	$F_{cal} = \dfrac{MSR}{MSE}$
Residual (Unexplained variation)	$n - 2$	SSE	MSE	
Total (Total variation)	$n - 1$	SST	MST	

The statistic F_{cal} in Table 2.1 is compared with the percentile of the Fisher's F-distribution with 1 and $n - 2$ degrees of freedom. This is considered to be evidence against H_0 if $F_{cal} > F_{(1,n-2)}$ for a certain level of significance. It is also possible to find p-values based on the F-distribution. In the case of SLRM, inference drawn from the F-test and the t-test are equivalent, since $F = t^2$; however, these tests are not equivalent in the case of multiple linear regression.

2.10 Coefficient of Determination R^2

The coefficient of determination R^2 is a measure of the goodness of fit of the model and is defined as

$$R^2 = \frac{\text{SSR}}{\text{SST}} \times 100\% \tag{2.20}$$

This coefficient determines the percentage of variation of the variable Y explained by the model. Another way to calculate R^2 is via the following formula:

$$R^2 = \left(1 - \frac{\text{SSE}}{\text{SST}}\right) \times 100\%$$

2.11 Pearson Correlation Coefficient

The Pearson correlation coefficient is an index indicating the degree of linear association between two continuous random variables. This coefficient is represented by ρ; its estimator is represented by $r = \hat{\rho}$. Its values range between -1.0 and 1.0. If r is close to 1.0 or to -1.0, there is a strong positive linear association (directly proportional) or negative (inversely proportional), respectively; values close to zero indicate little or no linear association. The mathematical expression for r is as follows:

$$r = \frac{\text{SSP}}{\sqrt{\text{SSX} \times \text{SST}}} \tag{2.21}$$

where

$\text{SSP} = \sum_{i=1}^{n} (y_i - \bar{y}) \times (x_i - \bar{x})$ denotes the total cross product of X and Y deviations.

$\text{SSX} = \sum_{i=1}^{n} (x_i - \bar{x})^2$ denotes the sum of squared deviations of X, which represents the total variation of X around its mean $(\bar{x})$.

An alternative way to calculate the Pearson correlation coefficient is from the square root of the coefficient of determination, using the sign of β_1, as previously estimated:

$$r = \text{sign}(\hat{\beta}_1) \times \sqrt{r^2}$$

To assess whether the Pearson correlation coefficient is different from zero (H_0: $\rho = 0$), with data from a random sample of size n, the following statistic is used:

$$t^* = \frac{r\sqrt{n-2}}{\sqrt{1-r^2}} \sim t_{n-2}$$

The Student's t-distribution with $n-2$ degrees of freedom is used to obtain the p-value. This test is equivalent to the t-test for assessing H_0: $\beta_1 = 0$, described in Section 2.9.1.

2.12 Estimation of Regression Line Values and Prediction

The goals of the SLRM can be summarized as follows:

i) Assess the linear association between X and Y. If they are significantly associated, how large is the change in the expected value of Y per unit of change in X?

ii) Predict the response variable for a given value of the predictor. For a point value of the predictor, we can estimate the conditional expected value of Y given a value of X, which is one of the values of the regression line, or we can estimate an actual value of Y given X. If the goal is the estimation of the conditional expected value of Y, then a confidence interval for the regression line is constructed. If the aim is to predict the actual value of the response variable, we obtain a prediction interval.

2.12.1 Confidence Interval for the Regression Line

The confidence interval to estimate the expected value of the regression line is as follows:

$$\hat{y}_k \pm t_{(n-2,(\alpha/2))} s_{Y|X} \sqrt{\frac{1}{n} + \frac{(x_k - \bar{x})^2}{\text{SSX}}} \tag{2.22}$$

where

$\hat{y}_k$ indicates the point estimation of the expected value for the kth observation.

$t_{(n-2,(\alpha/2))}$ indicates the value of the t-distribution with $n-2$ degrees of freedom and a significance level of α.

$s_{Y|X}$ indicates the standard error of the model.

x_k indicates the value of the predictor variable for the kth observation.

$\bar{x}$ indicates the average of the predictor variable.

SSX   indicates the sum of squares with respect to X.

2.12.2 Prediction Interval of Actual Values of the Response

The prediction interval to estimate the actual value Y is as follows:

$$\hat{y}_k \pm t_{(n-2,(\alpha/2))}s_{Y|X}\sqrt{1 + \frac{1}{n} + \frac{(x_k - \bar{x})^2}{\text{SSX}}} \tag{2.23}$$

The prediction intervals for actual values of Y are greater than the confidence intervals of the conditional expected value of Y, given that the standard error is greater when the unit in the part of the square root is included. This makes sense, since the interval is based on attempting to predict Y, a random variable (as opposed to estimating the expected value of Y given X, a nonrandom number).

2.13 Example

Waist circumference is a measure that has been used to identify individuals at increased risk for cardiovascular disease and type 2 diabetes. To identify people at increased risk of cardiovascular and metabolic diseases, standards have been established for waist circumference, blood pressure, triglycerides, high-density lipoprotein cholesterol (HDL-C), and fasting plasma glucose. For example, suppose that 20 adults between 21 and 79 years old have the data presented in Table 2.2 (Pérez et al., 2008):

i) What would be the linear regression model for this data set?
ii) What proportion of the variance in blood triglycerides level is explained by waist circumference?
iii) How large is the change in the expected value for blood triglycerides per unit of change in waist circumference? Is this change statistically significant?

First, we construct the scatter plot to assess the possible linear relationship between blood triglycerides and waist circumference (Figure 2.4). According to the scatter plot, there is a possible positive linear relationship between blood triglycerides and waist circumference for adults between 21 and 79 years old. Using STATA (v.14), the results of simple linear regression model are described in Table 2.3.

Table 2.2 Waist circumference and blood triglycerides of 20 adults between 21 and 79 years old.

Waist circumference (in.)	Triglycerides (mg/dl)	Waist circumference (in.)	Triglycerides (mg/dl)
32.95	28	40.5	90
33.0	40	43.5	107
33.5	50	42.0	109
33.5	61	39.4	111
34.5	66	40.2	112
37.0	70	44.9	119
35.0	79	43.5	121
36.85	85	44.8	130
36.45	87	41.5	149
40.65	89	45.0	159

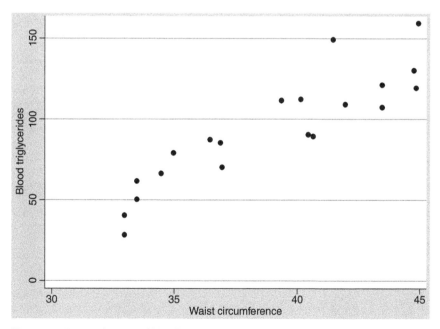

Figure 2.4 Scatter diagram of blood triglycerides and waist circumference.

Table 2.3 Analysis of the simple linear regression model.

```
reg trigl waist
    Source |       SS       df       MS        Number of obs   =        20
-------------+------------------------------   F(1, 18)        =     72.27
      Model |  18368.7813     1  18368.7813    Prob > F        =    0.0000
   Residual |  4575.01871    18  254.167706    R-squared       =    0.8006
-------------+------------------------------   Adj R-squared   =    0.7895
      Total |     22943.8    19  1207.56842    Root MSE        =    15.943
```

Trigl	Coefficient	Std. error	t	P > |t|	95% Confidence interval	
waist	7.23	0.85	8.5	0.000	5.45	9.02
_cons	−188.49	33.32	−5.66	0.000	−258.49	−118.50

The interpretation of Table 2.3 is as follows:

- Equation for the point estimate of the expected value

$$\hat{y}_{\text{trigl}|\text{waist}} = -188.5 + 7.23 \times \text{waist}$$

- Evaluation of $H_0 : \beta_1 = 0$

    $F_{\text{cal}} = 72.27$ (Variance ratio)

    Prob $> F = 0.0000$ (statistical packages often round off the results to a predefined number of digits)

    Decision: Evidence against H_0 ($p < 0.0001$)
    Conclusion: It is concluded that there is a linear relationship between blood triglycerides and waist circumference (*p*-value <0.0001). However, it remains to be answered if this a cause–effect relationship.
- The percentage of variation of blood triglycerides in adults between 21 and 79 years explained by the model is 80.06%.
- The point estimator of the variance of the triglycerides ($s^2_{\text{trigl}|\text{waist}}$) under the model is 254.17.

The point estimates of blood triglycerides (*triglexp*) for the observed waist circumferences are as follows:

waist	trigl	triglexp
32.95	28	49.81
33.0	40	50.18
33.5	50	53.79

waist	trigl	triglexp
33.5	61	53.79
34.5	66	61.02
37.0	70	79.11
35.0	79	64.64
36.85	85	78.02
36.5	87	75.13
40.7	89	105.50
40.5	90	104.42
43.5	107	126.12
42.0	109	115.27
39.4	111	96.46
40.2	112	102.25
44.9	119	136.24
43.5	121	126.12
44.8	130	135.52
41.5	149	111.65
45.0	159	136.96

According to the previous model, for an adult (or a group of adults) between 21 and 79 years old with a waist circumference of 42 in. the estimated expected value of blood triglycerides is 115.3 mg/dl.

2.14 Predictions

Once estimates of the SLRM are done, the following include some of the questions we can ask:

- What would be the estimate with 95% confidence of blood triglycerides expected for an adult between 21 and 79 years old with a waist circumference of 42 in.?
- What would be the estimate with 95% confidence of blood triglycerides expected for a group of adults between 21 and 79 years of age with a waist circumference of 42 in.?
- What would be the estimate with 95% confidence of blood triglycerides expected for an adult between 21 and 79 years old with a waist circumference of 38 in.?
- What would be the estimate with 95% confidence of blood triglycerides expected for a group of adults between 21 and 79 years of age with a waist circumference of 38 in.?

Two different aspects are included in the above questions. The value of the waist circumference of 42 in. forms part of the sample that was used to construct the SLRM, while the value 38 in. is not part of this. Let us see how we can solve these two situations in STATA.

2.14.1 Predictions with the Database Used by the Model

Based on the simple linear regression model, the standard errors will be, according to the aim of the regression line:

i) To estimate the expected value of Y

$$\text{error } 1 = s_{Y|X} \sqrt{\frac{1}{n} + \frac{(x_k - \bar{x})^2}{\text{SSX}}} \tag{2.24}$$

ii) For prediction of Y

$$\text{error } 2 = s_{Y|X} \sqrt{1 + \frac{1}{n} + \frac{(x_k - \bar{x})^2}{\text{SSX}}} \tag{2.25}$$

Using the SLRM for *trigl* described above, the values of *error 1* and *error 2* obtained in STATA are the following:

Observation	Waist (x)	trigl (y)	triglexp (ŷ)	error 1	error 2
1	32.95	28	49.81	6.22	17.11
2	33.0	40	50.18	6.18	17.10
3	33.5	50	53.79	5.84	16.98
4	33.5	61	53.79	5.84	16.98
5	34.5	66	61.02	5.19	16.77
6	37	70	79.11	3.93	16.42
7	35	79	64.64	4.89	16.68
8	36.85	85	78.02	3.98	16.43
9	36.45	87	75.13	4.14	16.47
10	40.65	89	105.50	3.85	16.40
11	40.5	90	104.42	3.81	16.39
12	43.5	107	126.12	5.27	16.79
13	42	109	115.27	4.42	16.54
14	39.4	111	96.46	3.59	16.34
15	40.2	112	102.25	3.72	16.37
16	44.9	119	136.24	6.20	17.11

Observation	Waist (x)	trigl (y)	triglexp ($\hat{y}$)	error 1	error 2
17	43.5	121	126.12	5.27	16.79
18	44.8	130	135.52	6.13	17.08
19	41.5	149	111.65	4.18	16.48
20	45	159	136.96	6.27	17.13

Then, the confidence interval of the expected value of Y and the prediction interval of an individual prediction will be defined as follows:

$$\left.\begin{array}{l} \inf = \hat{y}_k - t_{(n-2,(\alpha/2))} \times \text{error } 1 \\ \sup = \hat{y}_k + t_{(n-2,(\alpha/2))} \times \text{error } 1 \end{array}\right\} \quad \text{Confidence interval of the regression line}$$

$$\left.\begin{array}{l} \inf 1 = \hat{y}_k - t_{(n-2,(\alpha/2))} \times \text{error } 2 \\ \sup 1 = \hat{y}_k + t_{(n-2,(\alpha/2))} \times \text{error } 2 \end{array}\right\} \quad \begin{array}{l} \text{Prediction interval of an individual} \\ \text{prediction} \end{array}$$

In STATA, the results of these limits are as follows:

Observation	Waist	triglexp	inf	sup	inf 1	sup 1
1	32.95	49.81	36.76	62.87	13.86	85.76
2	33.0	50.18	37.19	63.16	14.25	86.10
3	33.5	53.79	41.53	66.06	18.12	89.46
4	33.5	53.79	41.53	66.06	18.12	89.46
5	34.5	61.02	50.12	71.93	25.80	96.25
6	37.0	79.11	70.86	87.35	44.61	113.60
7	35.0	64.64	54.37	74.91	29.61	99.68
8	36.85	78.02	69.65	86.39	43.50	112.54
9	36.45	75.13	66.42	83.83	40.52	109.74
10	40.65	105.50	97.41	113.60	71.05	139.96
11	40.5	104.42	96.42	112.41	69.98	138.85
12	43.5	126.12	115.04	137.19	90.84	161.39
13	42.0	115.27	105.99	124.55	80.51	150.02
14	39.4	96.46	88.93	104.00	62.13	130.79
15	40.2	102.25	94.43	110.07	67.85	136.64
16	44.9	136.24	123.21	149.27	100.30	172.18
17	43.5	126.12	115.04	137.19	90.84	161.39
18	44.8	135.52	122.63	148.40	99.63	171.40
19	41.5	111.65	102.87	120.43	77.02	146.28
20	45.0	136.96	123.79	150.14	100.97	172.96

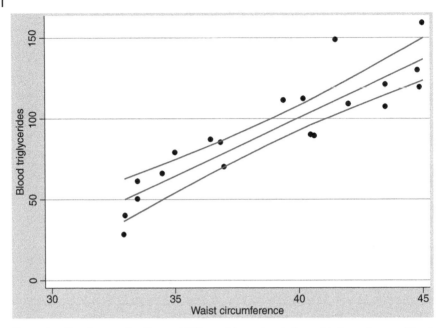

Figure 2.5 Fitted regression line and 95% confidence bands for waist circumference–blood triglycerides data.

The above data can be displayed with the construction of two graphs: one with the confidence bands of the regression line (Figure 2.5) and the other with individual prediction bands (Figure 2.6).

Using the above results, we conclude the following:

- The expected level of blood triglycerides for a group of adults between 21 and 79 years of age with a waist circumference of 42 in. is between 106.0 mg/dl and 124.6 mg/dl with a 95% confidence interval (95% CI: 106.0, 124.6).
- The predicted level of triglycerides in the blood for an adult between 21 and 79 years old with a waist circumference of 42 in. is between 80.5 and 150.0 mg/dl with a 95% prediction interval (95% CI: 80.5, 150.0).

2.14.2 Predictions with Data Not Used to Create the Model

The process of estimating the expected value of Y or predicting Y for values of the explanatory variable (or predictor) that are not part of the database used to create the model is similar to the above method but involves creating a new

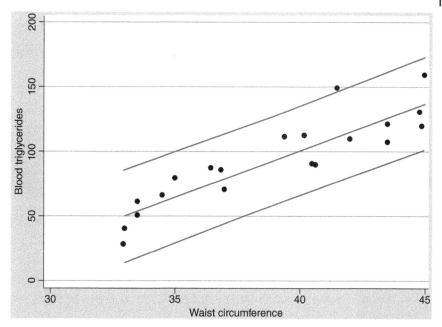

Figure 2.6 95% prediction bands for waist circumference–blood triglycerides data.

database containing only variable values of waist circumference to be estimated. To make this estimate, the steps in STATA are as follows:

i) Create the two databases (one with data to create the model and another to carry out predictions). The second database has one column that contains the values you want to use to perform the predictions, and the column name must be exactly the same name that was used in the first database.

ii) Run the regression model (using the command "reg").

iii) Use the command "clear" to inactivate the database that created the model.

iv) Read the second database (provided to carry out the predictions) with the command *use*.

v) Then use the command "predict" for the expected values and standard errors; for example,
   • to obtain the expected value predict yesp
   • to obtain the standard error of prediction lines predict eslp, stdp
   • to obtain the standard error of individual predictions predict esind, stdf

vi) Finally, use the command "gen" to construct confidence intervals, as follows:
   • Lower limit of the prediction lines with 95% confidence gen inf = yesp-invttail(18,0.025)*eslp

- Upper limit of the prediction lines with 95% confidence gen sup = yesp + invttail(18,0.025)*eslp
- Lower limit of a prediction with 95% confidence gen inf1 = yesp-invttail (18,0.025)*esind
- Upper limit of a prediction with 95% confidence gen sup1 = yesp + invttail(18,0.025)*esind

Using the previous model, the estimates of the expected level of blood triglycerides for a waist circumference of 38 in. are as follows:

Waist (x)	triglexp (ŷ)	inf	sup	inf 1	sup 1
38	86.3	78.66	94.01	51.97	120.70

These results are interpreted as follows:

- The expected level of blood triglycerides for a group of adults between 21 and 79 years of age with a waist circumference of 38 in. is between 78.66 and 94.01 mg/dl with 95% confidence.
- The predicted level of triglycerides in the blood for an adult between 21 and 79 years old with a waist circumference of 38 in. is between 51.97 and 120.70 mg/dl with 95% confidence.

Estimation of the response using predictor values outside the range of its observed values is known as extrapolation. Note that when we extrapolate, we are assuming the relationship is still linear.

2.14.3 Residual Analysis

In Section 2.4 the simple linear regression assumptions were presented. If these assumptions do not hold, hypothesis testing and confidence interval procedures may lead to the wrong conclusions. For example, if the assumption of independence of observations is invalid, t-statistics will tend to be higher than they should be, making it more likely to erroneously rejecting the null. Wrongfully treating the response variance as constant when it is not will lead to incorrect confidence interval bands, as would violating the normality assumption. The validity of the assumptions (and hence of the SLRM) can be assessed with the model residuals: the difference between the observed responses and the estimated responses according to the model. The difference between the observed blood triglycerides (trigl) and the expected blood triglycerides using the estimation of the SLRM (triglexp) are the residuals of the model in that example. The specific values of these residuals from the previous model are as follows:

waist	trigl	triglexp	res
33.0	28.0	49.81	−21.81
33.0	40.0	50.18	−10.18
33.5	50.0	53.79	−3.79
33.5	61.0	53.79	7.21
34.5	66.0	61.02	4.98
37.0	70.0	79.11	−9.11
35.0	79.0	64.64	14.36
36.9	85.0	78.02	6.98
36.5	87.0	75.13	11.87
40.7	89.0	105.50	−16.50
40.5	90.0	104.42	−14.42
43.5	107.0	126.12	−19.12
42.0	109.0	115.27	−6.27
39.4	111.0	96.46	14.54
40.2	112.0	102.25	9.75
44.9	119.0	136.24	−17.24
43.5	121.0	126.12	−5.12
44.8	130.0	135.52	−5.52
41.5	149.0	111.65	37.35
45.0	159.0	136.96	22.04

- *In the first adult:* The difference between the observed value of triglycerides (28) and the expected value of triglycerides (49.81) is −21.81.
- *In the 10th adult:* The difference between the observed value of triglycerides (89) and the expected value of triglycerides (105.50) is −16.50.
- *In the last adult:* The difference between the observed value of triglycerides (159) and the expected value of triglycerides (136.96) is 22.04.

The observed pattern in the residuals are difficult to evaluate with a table, particularly if we have a large number of subjects. Therefore, graphs are recommended to describe these residuals. One graph of use is the residual values versus the predictor values (Figure 2.7). The main assessment in this type of graph is to observe if the distribution of the residuals is uniform around zero to suggest constant variance. If for some X values the magnitude of the residuals are higher, or the magnitude of the residuals increases or decreases according to X values, then the variance is not constant. The graph is also used to check if the linear model assumption is appropriate: Any nonlinear pattern in this plot is indicative of a more complicated association between Y and X. Other plots, such as histograms and probability plots, are commonly used to assess the normal

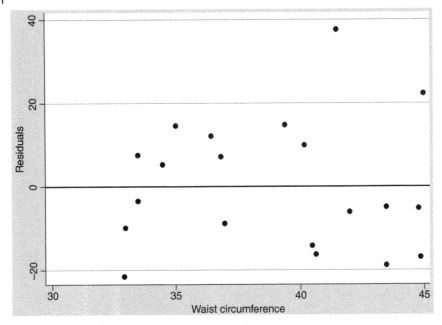

Figure 2.7 Residuals versus waist circumference plot.

distribution assumption. Although the residuals may be plotted against their order to evaluate the independence assumption, this plot often is not informative, and more advanced techniques are required. Residual plots can also be used to evaluate observations that individually have a large impact on the model results. However, since there is no way to determine when a residual is too large or too small, standardized residuals are used to evaluate the impact of individual observations. Standardized residuals are the residuals divided by their standard deviations. Any standardized residual that is too far above 3 or too far below −3 indicates that the observation requires a closer look as it may have a strong impact on the regression model results. Further strategies will be provided in Chapter 7 for assessing the adequacy of the linear regression model.

2.15 Conclusions

This chapter summarizes the use of SLRM. The expected values of a continuous random variable was modeled using a linear relationship with another continuous variable. The least-squares method for parameter estimation in this model was described. In addition, the methods for mean and individual predictions, based on this model, were presented using confidence and prediction intervals.

Finally, the procedures for assessing the basic assumptions of this model were explained using residual analysis. In the following chapters linear regression models will be extended and their application in epidemiology will be demonstrated.

Practice Exercise

In a hypothetical study blood samples were collected of 13 children infected with malaria. The following data represent the number of parasites (*number*) found in 1 ml of blood and the age of each infant under study:

Age	Number
12	730
8	143
16	2275
8	37
11	535
10	465
12	690
13	826
15	1340
14	1580
14	1340
15	1925
15	2662

a) Use a scatterplot to display the association between the natural logarithm of the number of parasites (response variable) and age (predictor). We recommend the use of the natural logarithm instead of the original scale because of the large variability in the data. To compute the natural logarithm of the variable number of parasites, use the *gen* and *log* commands as follows: *gen lnum = log(number)*.

b) Determine and interpret the Pearson correlation coefficient between *age* and *lnum*.

c) Determine the regression line of the natural logarithm of the number of parasites as a function of age and display the results in a graph.

d) Use a graph to display the behavior of the residuals against the fitted values. How do they behave around zero? Do you see any particular pattern?

e) Based on the logarithmic model, $\hat{y}_{\ln(\text{number})} = \hat{\beta}_0 + \hat{\beta}_1 \text{age}$, estimate the expected number of parasites in its original scale by age and display the results in a graph.

References

Bingham, N.H. and Fry, J.M. (2010) *Regression Linear Models in Statistics*. London, UK: Springer.

Gordis, L. (2014) *Epidemiology*, 5th edition. Philadelphia, PA: Elsevier Saunders.

Draper, N.R. and Smith, H. (1998) *Applied Regression Analysis*, 3rd edition. Hoboken, NJ: John Wiley & Sons, Inc.

Pérez, C., Guzmán, M., Ortiz, A.P., Estrella, M., Valle, Y., Pérez, N., Haddock, L., and Suárez, E. (2008) Prevalence of the metabolic syndrome in San Juan, Puerto Rico. *Ethn. Dis.*, **18**, 434–441.

3

Matrix Representation of the Linear Regression Model

Aim: Upon completing this chapter, the reader should be able to represent linear regression models using matrix notation and estimate the parameters for these models using STATA commands for matrix operations.

3.1 Introduction

Public health research involve situations with more than one independent or predictor variable. For example, if one wishes to predict the IQ of a child, some of the variables that can be used to obtain better estimates include parental education, maternal intelligence, and environmental and social factors. This chapter presents an extension of linear regression models to obtain predictions using more than one independent or predictor variable. These models are known as multiple linear regression models. Matrix notation will be used to facilitate the presentation of the estimation procedures and the evaluation of the parameters for these models.

3.2 Specific Objectives

The objectives of this chapter are as follows:

- Introduce the concept of multiple linear regression model using matrix theory.
- Know the assumptions of a multiple linear regression model in matrix form.
- Evaluate statistical hypothesis regarding the parameters of a multiple linear regression model through ANOVA.
- Estimate the percentage of variation of the response variable of the study explained by the multiple linear regression model.
- Estimate the expected value of the response variable using multiple linear regression models.

Applications of Regression Models in Epidemiology, First Edition. Erick Suárez,
Cynthia M. Pérez, Roberto Rivera, and Melissa N. Martínez.
© 2017 John Wiley & Sons, Inc. Published 2017 by John Wiley & Sons, Inc.

- Evaluate the behavior of residuals in a multiple linear regression model.
- Apply a multiple linear regression model to study a public health problem.

3.3 Definition

3.3.1 Matrix

A matrix is a set of numbers arranged in rectangular shape, where the numbers are located by a row (or line) and a column. For example,

	Column 1	Column 2
Row 1	1	3
Row 2	10	-9
Row 3	11	7

Matrices are usually identified by a bold capital letter and framed by a parenthesis or brace. For example,

$$\mathbf{A} = \begin{bmatrix} 1 & 3 \\ 10 & -9 \\ 11 & 7 \end{bmatrix}$$

The data set to evaluate a regression model can be organized into a matrix, where rows represent subjects and columns identify the study variables.

The *dimensions of a matrix* are defined by the number of rows and columns. In the above example, the dimensions would be 3×2. An abstract form of representing a matrix is

$$\mathbf{A}_{rxc} = \{a_{ij}\}, \quad \text{for} \quad i = 1, \ldots, r; \quad j = 1, \ldots, c$$

A *square matrix* $\mathbf{A}_{rxc}$ is one whose number of rows equals the number of columns, that is, $r = c$.

A *column vector* is a matrix with dimension $r \times 1$.

A *row vector* is a matrix with dimension $1 \times c$.

A *transposed matrix* is a matrix that is identified by A' and obtained by interchanging the rows and columns of the matrix $\mathbf{A}$. The element a_{ij} of the matrix $\mathbf{A}$ will be the element a_{ji} in the transposed matrix A'.

3.4 Matrix Representation of a SLRM

The value of the response variable for an individual may be expressed by

$$y_i = \beta_0 + \beta_1 x_i + e_i$$

Therefore, for all study subjects combined, the random variable Y under study can be represented as a column vector as follows:

$$\mathbf{Y}_{n \times 1} = \begin{bmatrix} y_1 \\ \vdots \\ y_n \end{bmatrix}, \mathbf{Y}'_{1 \times n} = \begin{bmatrix} y_1 & \cdots & y_n \end{bmatrix}$$

Likewise, the independent variable values can be represented as follows:

$$\mathbf{X}_{n \times 2} = \begin{bmatrix} 1 & x_1 \\ \vdots & \vdots \\ 1 & x_n \end{bmatrix}$$

The first column of 1's is used to identify the coefficient β_0, which is multiplied by the unit number. The second column is associated with the values of the independent variable X, which will affect values of Y in conjunction with the coefficient β_1. The subscript in the variable X indicates the value of this variable for subject i.

3.5 Matrix Arithmetic

3.5.1 Addition and Subtraction of Matrices

If $\mathbf{A}$ and $\mathbf{B}$ are two matrices of the same dimension, then

$$\mathbf{A}_{k \times m} \pm \mathbf{B}_{k \times m} = \left\{ a_{ij} \pm b_{ij} \right\} = \mathbf{C}_{k \times m}$$

The result will be another matrix with the same dimension of $\mathbf{A}$ and $\mathbf{B}$. Note that matrices that are being added or subtracted must have the same dimensions. For example,

$$\text{if } \mathbf{A} = \begin{bmatrix} 1 & -1 \\ 2 & 4 \\ 5 & 6 \end{bmatrix} \quad \text{and} \quad \mathbf{B} = \begin{bmatrix} 1 & 5 \\ 3 & -3 \\ -7 & 0 \end{bmatrix}, \quad \text{then} \quad \mathbf{A} + \mathbf{B} = \mathbf{C} = \begin{bmatrix} 2 & 4 \\ 5 & 1 \\ -2 & 6 \end{bmatrix}$$

The model $y_i = \beta_0 + \beta_1 x_i + e_i$, represents

$$
\begin{aligned}
y_1 &= \beta_0 + \beta_1 x_1 + e_1 \\
y_2 &= \beta_0 + \beta_1 x_2 + e_2 \\
\vdots \quad & \qquad \vdots \\
y_n &= \beta_0 + \beta_1 x_n + e_n
\end{aligned}
$$

This can be also represented as the sum of two matrices:

$$\begin{bmatrix} y_1 \\ y_2 \\ \vdots \\ y_n \end{bmatrix} = \begin{bmatrix} \beta_0 + \beta_1 x_1 \\ \beta_0 + \beta_1 x_2 \\ \vdots \\ \beta_0 + \beta_1 x_n \end{bmatrix} + \begin{bmatrix} e_1 \\ e_2 \\ \vdots \\ e_n \end{bmatrix} \tag{3.1}$$

That is, the matrix of the observed values $\{\mathbf{Y}_{nx1}\}$ equals the expected value of Y $\{\mathbf{X}\boldsymbol{\beta}_{nx1}\}$ plus an error matrix $\{\mathbf{e}_{nx1}\}$.

3.6 Matrix Multiplication

Multiplication of a matrix by a constant K. To multiply a matrix by a constant K, the constant multiplies each matrix entry. So,

$$\text{if } \mathbf{A} = \begin{bmatrix} 2 & 1 \\ 3 & -5 \end{bmatrix} \text{ and } K = 3, \text{ then } 3\mathbf{A} = \begin{bmatrix} 3(2) & 3(1) \\ 3(3) & 3(-5) \end{bmatrix} = \begin{bmatrix} 6 & 3 \\ 9 & -15 \end{bmatrix}$$

Multiplication of two matrices. For matrix multiplication the number of columns of the first matrix must be equal to the number of rows in the second matrix. The result of this multiplication is a matrix of dimension equal to the number of rows in the first matrix by the number of columns in the second matrix:

$$\mathbf{A}_{mxn}\mathbf{B}_{nxk} = \mathbf{C}_{mxk}$$

In matrix algebra, $\mathbf{AB} = \mathbf{BA}$ is not necessarily true. To multiply two matrices, the recommended steps are as follows:

i) Identify the dimension of the resulting matrix of the product of two matrices.
ii) Multiply each element of a row in the first matrix by the elements of each column of the second matrix.
iii) For each product of rows and columns, calculate the sum.
iv) This sum defines each element of the resulting matrix of the matrix product.

For example, let $\mathbf{A} = \begin{bmatrix} 1 & -3 & 2 \\ 0 & 5 & 8 \end{bmatrix}$ and $= \begin{bmatrix} 3 \\ 5 \\ 2 \end{bmatrix}$. Then $\mathbf{AB} = \mathbf{C}$ is calculated as follows:

$$\mathbf{A}_{2x3}\mathbf{B}_{3x1} = \begin{bmatrix} (1 \times 3) + (-3 \times 5) + (2 \times 2) \\ (0 \times 3) + (5 \times 5) + (8 \times 2) \end{bmatrix} = \begin{bmatrix} -8 \\ 41 \end{bmatrix} = \mathbf{C}_{2x1}$$

Let β and X be the following matrices:

$$\beta = \begin{bmatrix} \beta_0 \\ \beta_1 \end{bmatrix}$$

$$X = \begin{bmatrix} 1 & x_1 \\ 1 & x_2 \\ \vdots & \vdots \\ 1 & x_n \end{bmatrix}$$

the product $X\beta$ is a matrix of dimension $n \times 1$:

$$X\beta = \begin{bmatrix} 1 & x_1 \\ 1 & x_2 \\ \vdots & \vdots \\ 1 & x_n \end{bmatrix} \begin{bmatrix} \beta_0 \\ \beta_1 \end{bmatrix} = \begin{bmatrix} \beta_0 + \beta_1 x_1 \\ \beta_0 + \beta_1 x_2 \\ \vdots \\ \beta_0 + \beta_1 x_n \end{bmatrix} \tag{3.2}$$

If β is the coefficient matrix of a SLRM and X is the matrix of the predictor variable, the matrix $X\beta$ is the column vector of the expected values of Y (since the model errors are assumed to have an expected value of zero). Other examples of products of matrices in regression are as follows:

i) $$Y'Y = \begin{bmatrix} y_1 \cdots y_n \end{bmatrix} \begin{bmatrix} y_1 \\ \vdots \\ y_n \end{bmatrix} = \begin{bmatrix} y_1^2 + y_2^2 + \cdots + y_n^2 \end{bmatrix} = \begin{bmatrix} \sum_{i=1}^{n} y_i^2 \end{bmatrix} \tag{3.3}$$

ii) $$X'X = \begin{bmatrix} 1 & \cdots & 1 \\ x_1 & \cdots & x_n \end{bmatrix} \begin{bmatrix} 1 & x_1 \\ \vdots & \vdots \\ 1 & x_n \end{bmatrix} = \begin{bmatrix} n & \sum_{i=1}^{n} x_i \\ \sum_{i=1}^{n} x_i & \sum_{i=1}^{n} x_i^2 \end{bmatrix} \tag{3.4}$$

iii) $$X'Y = \begin{bmatrix} 1 & \cdots & 1 \\ x_1 & \cdots & x_n \end{bmatrix} \begin{bmatrix} y_1 \\ \vdots \\ y_2 \end{bmatrix} = \begin{bmatrix} \sum_{i=1}^{n} y_i \\ \sum_{i=1}^{n} x_i y_i \end{bmatrix} \tag{3.5}$$

3.7 Special Matrices

Other matrices useful in the linear regression analysis are as follows:

- **Symmetric Matrix:** A square matrix A is a symmetric matrix if $A = A'$. That is, $[a_{ij}] = [a_{ji}]$ for all i, j.
  Note: Verify that the matrix $(X'X)$ used in simple linear regression is a symmetric matrix.

- **Diagonal Matrix:** A square matrix **A** is a diagonal matrix if all entries other than those on the main diagonal are zeros. That is, $[a_{ij}] = 0$ for all $i \neq j$.
- **Identity Matrix:** An identity matrix is a diagonal matrix where $[a_{ii}] = 1$ for all i.
  Note: Any matrix $\mathbf{A}_{n \times n}$ multiplied by an identity matrix $\mathbf{I}_{n \times n}$ results in the same matrix. That is, $\mathbf{IA} = \mathbf{AI} = \mathbf{A}$.
- **Scalar Matrix:** A scalar matrix is a diagonal matrix where $[a_{ii}] = \lambda$, λ being a constant. If $\lambda = 1$, the resulting matrix is the identity matrix.
- **Null Vector:** A null vector is a row or column vector where all entries are zeros (also known as zero vector).

3.8 Linear Dependence

A matrix can be viewed as a set of column vectors as is shown below:

$$\mathbf{A} = \begin{bmatrix} 1 & 2 & 5 & 1 \\ 2 & 2 & 10 & 6 \\ 3 & 4 & 15 & 1 \end{bmatrix} = \left[\begin{pmatrix} 1 \\ 2 \\ 3 \end{pmatrix} \begin{pmatrix} 2 \\ 2 \\ 4 \end{pmatrix} \begin{pmatrix} 5 \\ 10 \\ 15 \end{pmatrix} \begin{pmatrix} 1 \\ 6 \\ 1 \end{pmatrix} \right]$$

Linear dependence exists between columns when we have a set of scalars $(\lambda_1, \lambda_2, \dots, \lambda_p)$, not all equal to zero, so that:

$$\lambda_1 C_1 + \lambda_2 C_2 + \cdots + \lambda_p C_p = 0 \tag{3.6}$$

If this relation is satisfied only when all $\lambda_i's$ are equal to zero, then the columns are *linearly independent*. One way of detecting linear dependence is when one column is a multiple of another column. For example, in the above matrix **A**, $C_3 = 5\,C_1$, therefore linear dependence exists between these columns.

3.9 Rank of a Matrix

The rank of a matrix is the maximum number of columns that are linearly independent. The rank of **A**, denoted by rank[**A**], is always less than or equal to the minimum number of rows or columns of the matrix:

$$\text{rank}[A] \leq \min(r, c)$$

3.10 Inverse Matrix $[\mathbf{A}^{-1}]$

The inverse matrix of **A**, identified by $\mathbf{A}^{-1}$, is defined only for square matrices. However, there are square matrices with no inverse. The inverse of a matrix $\mathbf{A}_{r \times r}$ exists as long as **A** is a matrix of full rank; that is, the rank of the matrix is r. A matrix is *nonsingular* when its rank is r. If the rank is less than r, the matrix is *singular* and has no inverse.

Method for finding the inverse of a 2×2 matrix

Suppose that $\mathbf{A} = \begin{bmatrix} a & b \\ c & d \end{bmatrix}$. The inverse of $\mathbf{A}$ is given by

$$\mathbf{A}^{-1} = \frac{1}{D}\begin{bmatrix} d & -b \\ -c & a \end{bmatrix} = \begin{bmatrix} d/D & -b/D \\ -c/D & a/D \end{bmatrix}$$

where $D = ad - bc$ is called the determinant of matrix $\mathbf{A}$.

To verify that the inverse of a matrix is correct, the following condition must be met:

$$\mathbf{A}\mathbf{A}^{-1} = \mathbf{A}^{-1}\mathbf{A} = \mathbf{I}$$

where $\mathbf{I}$ is an identity matrix of the same order as $\mathbf{A}$.

Verify that $\begin{bmatrix} d/D & -b/D \\ -c/D & a/D \end{bmatrix}$ is the inverse of $\begin{bmatrix} a & b \\ c & d \end{bmatrix}$, that is, show that

$$\begin{bmatrix} a & b \\ c & d \end{bmatrix}\begin{bmatrix} d/D & -b/D \\ -c/D & a/D \end{bmatrix} = \begin{bmatrix} 1 & 0 \\ 0 & 1 \end{bmatrix}$$

Method for finding the inverse of a 3×3 matrix

Suppose that $\mathbf{B} = \begin{bmatrix} a & b & c \\ d & e & f \\ g & h & k \end{bmatrix}$. The inverse of $\mathbf{B}$ is given by

$$\mathbf{B}^{-1} = \begin{bmatrix} A & B & C \\ D & E & F \\ G & H & K \end{bmatrix}$$

where

$$A = (ek - fh)/Z \quad D = -(bk - ch)/Z \quad G = (bf - ce)/Z$$
$$B = -(dk - fg)/Z \quad E = (ak - cg)/Z \quad H = -(af - cd)/Z$$
$$C = (dh - eg)/Z \quad F = -(ah - bg)/Z \quad K = (ae - bd)/Z$$

and

$$Z = a(ek - fh) - b(dk - fg) + c(dh - eg) \text{ is the determinant of the matrix } \mathbf{B}.$$

3.11 Application of an Inverse Matrix in a SLRM

Given $(\mathbf{X}'\mathbf{X}) = \begin{bmatrix} n & \sum_{i=1}^{n} x_i \\ \sum_{i=1}^{n} x_i & \sum_{i=1}^{n} x_i^2 \end{bmatrix}$, its inverse is given by the following matrix:

$$(\mathbf{X}'\mathbf{X})^{-1} = \begin{bmatrix} \dfrac{\sum_{i=1}^{n} x_i^2}{D} & -\dfrac{\sum_{i=1}^{n} x_i}{D} \\ -\dfrac{\sum_{i=1}^{n} x_i}{D} & \dfrac{n}{D} \end{bmatrix} \tag{3.7}$$

where D represents the determinant of the matrix $(\mathbf{X}'\mathbf{X})$, calculated using the following formula:

$$D = n\left(\sum_{i=1}^{n} x_i^2\right) - \left(\sum_{i=1}^{n} x_i\right)\left(\sum_{i=1}^{n} x_i\right) = n\left(\sum_{i=1}^{n} x_i^2 - \frac{\left(\sum_{i=1}^{n} x_i\right)^2}{n}\right) = n\sum_{i=1}^{n} (x_i - \bar{x})^2$$

3.12 Estimation of β Parameters in a SLRM

The representation of a SLRM in matrix form is given as

$$\mathbf{Y}_{n\times1} = \mathbf{X}_{n\times2}\boldsymbol{\beta}_{2\times1} + \mathbf{e}_{n\times1} \tag{3.8}$$

It is common to use this matrix representation without subscripts, that is,

$$\mathbf{Y} = \mathbf{X}\boldsymbol{\beta} + \mathbf{e}$$

To estimate the $\boldsymbol{\beta}$'s parameters by the method of least squares, we need to minimize the following function:

$$S = \sum_{i=1}^{n} e_i^2$$

The matrix form of this function is $S = \mathbf{e}'\mathbf{e}$, $\mathbf{e}$ being the vector of residuals. Thus,

$$S = (\mathbf{Y} - \mathbf{X}\boldsymbol{\beta})'(\mathbf{Y} - \mathbf{X}\boldsymbol{\beta}) \tag{3.9}$$

The following equations can be obtained by doing a bit of vector algebra (Draper and Smith, 1998):

$$S = Y'Y - \beta'X'Y - Y'X\beta + \beta'X'X\beta = Y'Y - 2\beta'X'Y + \beta'X'X\beta$$

The values of the β_i' coefficients that minimize S will be the estimators of these coefficients. As a result of this minimization process using the least-squares method, the following equation is obtained, known as the *regression normal equation* in matrix form:

$$X'X\beta = X'Y \tag{3.10}$$

In the case of simple linear regression, this matrix is

$$\begin{bmatrix} n & \sum x_i \\ \sum x_i & \sum x_i^2 \end{bmatrix} \begin{bmatrix} \beta_0 \\ \beta_1 \end{bmatrix} = \begin{bmatrix} \sum x_i \\ \sum x_i y_i \end{bmatrix}$$

When $(X'X)^{-1}$ exists, then

$$(X'X)^{-1}(X'X)\beta = (X'X)^{-1}X'Y$$

The vector $\hat{\beta}$ defines the estimators of the $\beta_i's$ coefficients:

$$\hat{\beta} = (X'X)^{-1}X'Y = \begin{bmatrix} \hat{\beta}_0 \\ \hat{\beta}_1 \end{bmatrix} \tag{3.11}$$

The variance of these estimators is obtained from the diagonal values of the following matrix:

$$Var\left(\hat{\beta}\right) = \sigma^2 (X'X)^{-1}$$

where σ^2 represents the variance of the regression errors. In practice σ^2 is estimated by MSE, the mean square error of the regression model. The matrix product obtained is known as the variance and covariance matrix of the estimators β_0 and β_1. In the case of simple linear regression, this matrix is expressed as follows:

$$Var\left(\hat{\beta}\right) = \sigma^2 (X'X)^{-1} = \begin{bmatrix} Var(\hat{\beta}_0) & Cov(\hat{\beta}_0, \hat{\beta}_1) \\ Cov(\hat{\beta}_0, \hat{\beta}_1) & Var(\hat{\beta}_1) \end{bmatrix} \tag{3.12}$$

To obtain the standard errors of $\hat{\beta}_0$ and $\hat{\beta}_1$, the square root of the diagonal values of the variance and covariance matrix is calculated as follows:

$$se(\hat{\beta}_i) = \left(Var(\hat{\beta}_i)\right)^{1/2}$$

3.13 Multiple Linear Regression Model (MLRM)

Suppose there is a total of p predictors variables and n observations. The MLRM is represented as follows:

$$y_i = \beta_0 + \beta_1 x_{i1} + \beta_2 x_{i2} + \cdots + \beta_p x_{ip} + e_i \tag{3.13}$$

for $i = 1, \ldots, n$.

This model can be expressed in matrix notation as

$$Y = X\beta + e$$

where

$$Y = \begin{bmatrix} y_1 \\ y_2 \\ \vdots \\ y_n \end{bmatrix} \quad X = \begin{bmatrix} 1 & x_{11} & x_{12} & \cdots & x_{1p} \\ 1 & x_{21} & x_{22} & \cdots & x_{2p} \\ \vdots & \vdots & \vdots & \vdots & \vdots \\ 1 & x_{n1} & x_{n2} & \cdots & x_{np} \end{bmatrix} \quad \beta = \begin{bmatrix} \beta_0 \\ \beta_1 \\ \vdots \\ \beta_p \end{bmatrix} \quad e = \begin{bmatrix} e_1 \\ e_2 \\ \vdots \\ e_n \end{bmatrix}$$

In general, Y is a vector of observations $(n \times 1)$, X is a matrix $(n \times (p + 1))$ of independent variables, β is a vector of regression coefficients $((p + 1) \times 1)$, and e is a vector of random errors $(n \times 1)$. The first column of X represents the intercept of the model, while the other columns represent each predictor.

3.14 Interpretation of the Coefficients in a MLRM

When the predictors of the MLRM are uncorrelated, the β_i coefficient measures the expected change in the variable Y per unit change in the predictor X_i, when all other predictors are held constant. If β_i is positive, the expected value of the response variable increases in the number of units indicated by the coefficient; if the coefficient is negative, the expected value of the response variable decreases. One common problem in MLRM is that predictors are often correlated, so it is advisable to examine their correlations, assess the changes in the regression coefficients according to whether other variables are included or excluded from the model, and employ collinearity diagnostics to identify multicollinearity (Jewell, 2004). We turn to that topic in Section 3.19.

3.15 ANOVA in a MLRM

To assess whether at least one of the β_i coefficients, for $i > 0$, is nonzero, it is necessary to carry out an ANOVA. To calculate the sum of squares in this analysis, the following expressions are used:

Sum of squares due to independent variables in regression, with p degrees of freedom:

$$SSR = \hat{\beta}' X' Y - n\overline{Y}^2 \tag{3.14}$$

Sum of squares due to error with $n - p - 1$ degrees of freedom:

$$SSE = Y'Y - \hat{\beta}' X'Y \tag{3.15}$$

Total sum of squares with $n - 1$ degrees of freedom:

$$SST = Y'Y - n\overline{Y}^2 \tag{3.16}$$

where n is the sample size and p is the number of predictor variables. The total sum of squares is decomposed in terms of the independent components SSR and SSE:

$$SST = SSR + SSE$$

Under the null hypothesis, an unbiased estimator of the response variable variance can be obtained based on either SSR or SSE. Specifically, $MSR = SSR/p$ and $MSE = SSE/(n - p - 1)$, as described in Table 3.1. When the null hypothesis is not true, then MSR is biased as it will overestimate the variance of the response variable.

It can be shown that the calculated value of the test statistic, F_{cal}, in Table 3.1 will follow an F-distribution with p numerator degrees of freedom and $n - p - 1$ denominator degrees of freedom. If F_{cal} is greater than the critical value $F_{(p, n-p-1)}$ for a given significance level, we conclude that there is evidence against H_0. Equivalently, statistical software often obtains a p-value based on F_{cal}. Depending on the number of predictor variables in the model, one can consider the following hypotheses:

- For a SLRM, $y_i = \beta_0 + \beta_1 x + e_i$, the hypotheses are $H_0 : \beta_1 = 0$ versus $H_a : \beta_1 \neq 0$. Rejecting H_0 means that there is a linear relationship between the response variable and the predictor variable.
- In the case of the MLRM, $y_i = \beta_0 + \beta_1 x_1 + \beta_2 x_2 + \cdots + \beta_p x_p + e_i$, the hypotheses are $H_0 : \beta_1 = \beta_2 = \cdots = \beta_p = 0$ versus $H_a :$ At least one of the regression coefficients is nonzero. Rejecting H_0 means that at least one of the predictor variables of the model can be used to explain the variation of the variable **Y**. However, the hypothesis test does not tell us which coefficients are different to zero. We turn to that topic in the next chapter.

Table 3.1 ANOVA for a multiple linear regression model.

Source of variation	Degrees of freedom	Sum of squares	Mean squares	Statistic F_{cal}
Regression (explained variation)	p	SSR	$MSR = SSR/p$	$F_{cal} = \dfrac{MSR}{MSE}$
Residual (unexplained variation)	$n - p - 1$	SSE	$MSE = SSE/(n - p - 1)$	
Total (total variation)	$n - 1$	SST		

3.16 Using Indicator Variables *(Dummy Variables)*

Another important application of a regression model is to use the coefficients as measures to identify differences in the expected value of a continuous random variable between two or more groups of study. That is, a regression model when the predictor is a categorical variable. For example, assuming that there are three groups of interest (children, adolescents, and adults), and we want to compare the expected levels of hemoglobin in these groups, the initial model would be

$$\mathbf{Y}_{ij} = \boldsymbol{\mu}_j + \mathbf{e}_{ij} \tag{3.17}$$

where $\mathbf{Y}_{ij}$ indicates the value of the random variable hemoglobin levels in the subject i that belongs to group j (e.g., $j=1$ children, $j=2$ adolescents, and $j=3$ adults), e_{ij} indicates the difference between the observed value of $\mathbf{Y}_{ij}$ and the expected value of the random variable $\mathbf{Y}$ in the group j (μ_j).

This model can be redefined or reparametrized as follows:

$$\mathbf{Y}_{ij} = \boldsymbol{\mu}_j + 0 + \mathbf{e}_{ij} = \boldsymbol{\mu}_j + (\boldsymbol{\mu}_1 - \boldsymbol{\mu}_1) + \mathbf{e}_{ij}$$

$$\mathbf{Y}_{ij} = \boldsymbol{\mu}_1 + \left(\boldsymbol{\mu}_j - \boldsymbol{\mu}_1\right) + \mathbf{e}_{ij}$$

$$\mathbf{Y}_{ij} = \boldsymbol{\mu}_1 + \boldsymbol{\delta}_j + \mathbf{e}_{ij}$$

where $\delta_j = \mu_j - \mu_1$ indicates the difference between the expected value for the group j and the first group, denoted as the reference group. This is also identified as the effect of the group j. The reference group could be defined based on any group; usually computer programs take as a reference group the one that has the lowest coded value or greater coded value. When compared groups represent all possible groups, or when they represent groups of interest, the δ_js are constants and are defined as fixed effects.

Therefore, the expected value of $\mathbf{Y}_{ij}$, assuming fixed effects, is $\mu_{Y_j} = \mu_1 + \delta_j$. This representation can be expressed as a linear regression model as follows:

$$\mu_{Y_j} = \mu_1 + \delta_j = \mu_1 + \delta_1^* Z_1 + \delta_2^* Z_2 + \delta_3^* Z_3 \tag{3.18}$$

where

$Z_1 = 1$ if the expected value is of a child, $Z_1 = 0$ if another group.
$Z_2 = 1$ if the expected value is of an adolescent, $Z_2 = 0$ if another group.
$Z_3 = 1$ if the expected value is of an adult, $Z_3 = 0$ if another group.

Letting $\delta_1 = 0$ when the first group is the reference group, the model is defined as

$$\mu_{Y_j} = \mu_1 + \delta_j^* Z_j$$

for $j = 2, 3$

The expression Z_j is identified as an indicator variable or *dummy variable* that has only two values: 0 and 1. If one of the Z_j is equal to 1, the others are 0. To estimate the values of the δ'_j effects, use the matrix X of a linear regression model as defined in Section 3.12. For example, assuming three groups, the matrix is defined as follows:

	Constant	Group 2	Group 3	
	1	0	0	
	1	0	0	
	1	0	0	Group 1
	1	0	0	
	1	0	0	
	1	0	0	
$X =$	1	1	0	
	1	1	0	
	1	1	0	Group 2
	1	1	0	
	1	1	0	
	1	0	1	
	1	0	1	Group 3
	1	0	1	
	1	0	1	
	1	0	1	

That is, a column with 1's and two columns of 1's or 0's, depending on the group to which the subject belongs. Note that no column for group 1 was used since its value (1 or 0) can be deduced from the other two columns. Furthermore, including it would lead to the columns being linearly dependent and hence to noninvertibility of $(X'X)$. If we cannot obtain the inverse of $(X'X)$, we cannot obtain unique least-squares estimates of the regression coefficients. Assuming that the values of the transpose of Y are equal to

$$Y' = \{10, 11, 9, 8, 10, 11, 12, 13, 12, 13, 11, 14, 15, 16, 13, 14\}$$

the data would be as follows:

c	z1	z2	y
1	0	0	10
1	0	0	11

c	z1	z2	y
1	0	0	9
1	0	0	8
1	0	0	10
1	0	0	11
1	1	0	12
1	1	0	13
1	1	0	12
1	1	0	13
1	1	0	11
1	0	1	14
1	0	1	15
1	0	1	16
1	0	1	13
1	0	1	14

Once these data are defined, the estimation of the group effects, δ_js, can be obtained the same way as the coefficients of a multiple linear regression model. Using the previous data, the results of these estimations are

$$\hat{\delta} = (\mathbf{X}'\mathbf{X})^{-1}\mathbf{X}'\mathbf{Y} = \begin{bmatrix} \overline{Y}_1 \\ \hat{\delta}_2 \\ \hat{\delta}_3 \end{bmatrix} = \begin{bmatrix} \overline{Y}_1 \\ \overline{Y}_2 - \overline{Y}_1 \\ \overline{Y}_3 - \overline{Y}_1 \end{bmatrix} = \begin{bmatrix} 9.83 \\ 2.36 \\ 4.56 \end{bmatrix}$$

The effect $\hat{\delta}_2 = 2.36$ indicates the estimated difference in the mean of Y in group 2 (adolescents) and the mean of Y in group 1 (children). The effect $\hat{\delta}_3 = 4.56$ indicates the estimated difference in the mean of Y in group 3 (adults) and the mean of Y in group 1 (children). Just as the standard errors (se) of the coefficients of the linear regression model were obtained, the standard errors of the effects δ can be estimated with the expression $\widehat{\text{Var}}(\hat{\delta}) = \text{MSE}(\mathbf{X}'\mathbf{X})^{-1}$. With the data above, the standard error would be $\text{se}(\hat{\delta}_j) = 0.65$ for both effects. Assuming normally distributed regression errors, the ratio of the estimates of the effects δ_j and their corresponding standard errors can be used to evaluate individually the statistical significance of a specific effect; however, the ANOVA results will assess simultaneously these effects, $H_0 : \delta_2 = \delta_3 = 0$. As stated in Section 2.9, for SLRM there are two equivalent hypothesis tests: ANOVA and t-tests. ANOVA answers the question: "Is the model worthwhile?". On the other hand, the t-tests answers the question: "Is the predictor important?". Since in SLRM there is only one predictor, the answers to these questions are equivalent.

However, in the case of MLRM, the model may be worthwhile, but with only some predictors being important. To avoid incurring in type I errors, it is best to perform an ANOVA first. If the null hypothesis is rejected, then at least one of the predictors is linearly related to the response variable. To determine which predictors are important, t-tests are an alternative as long as there are not too many predictors to test. Otherwise, other strategies may be needed. We discuss some of these strategies in the following chapters.

3.17 Polynomial Regression Models

There are special cases of a MLRM where independent variables may not be linearly associated with Y. For example, the simplest case would be the following model:

$$Y_i = \beta_0 + \beta_1 x_i + \beta_2 x_i^2 + e_i \tag{3.19}$$

This expression corresponds to a second-degree polynomial model, since it contains an independent variable expressed as a term to the first power (x_i) and a term expressed to the second power (x_i^2). For example, a fitted second-degree polynomial model is shown in Figure 3.1.

A third-degree polynomial model with two independent variables can be expressed by the equation $Y_i = \beta_0 + \beta_1 x_i + \beta_2 x_i^2 + \beta_3 x_i^3 + e_i$ (see Figure 3.2).

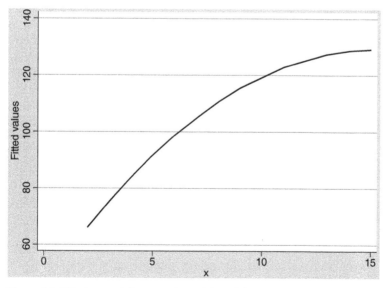

Figure 3.1 Fitted second-degree polynomial model.

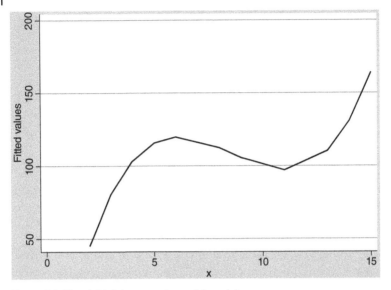

Figure 3.2 Fitted third-degree polynomial model.

These models can be used to describe a curvilinear rather than a linear relationship between the dependent (Y) and independent (X) variables. The main concern in using these models is when making predictions outside the range of values of the independent variables used to construct the model, something that must also be considered when the model describes a linear association between Y and X. Moreover, columns of Xs are now dependent and therefore coefficient estimates become less stable. In models with higher degree polynomial models, changes in the direction of the association between Y and X occur, while the expected value of Y continues to increase. That is, $E(Y_i)$ shows an increasing trend but at certain points Y and X are negatively correlated due to the power functions included in the model (Kutner et al., 2004).

3.18 Centering

The interpretation of the regression coefficients is sensitive to the scale of measurement of the explanatory variables and no coefficient is more affected by this than the intercept. This is why up to this point no attempt has been made to make inferences about the intercept. Recall that, mathematically, the estimated intercept is the value of the fitted value of the main outcome when all explanatory variables are zero. But in many real life situations, explanatory variables cannot be equal to zero. To facilitate interpretation of the intercept in a linear regression model, it is advisable to transform the X values based on the difference of each value from its mean: $X_i - \overline{X}_i$. This transformation is known as *centering.* As a result of centering, the estimator of the intercept coefficient is equal to the average of the dependent variable $\left(\hat{\beta}_0 = \overline{Y}\right)$. This process does not affect the estimates of the coefficients associated with the independent variables. Another advantage of centering the independent variables is that it reduces the impact of multicollinearity and also helps in the interpretation of interactions, two concepts that are discussed in the following section. Another similar technique is standardization, which consists of centering followed by dividing by the standard deviation of the respective explanatory variable. This technique makes regression coefficients more comparable among models.

3.19 Multicollinearity

One problem in the estimation of regression coefficients, β_i, is that correlations may exist between independent variables. When there is a perfect correlation between two independent variables, then one independent variable is a linear combination of another independent variable. Recall that perfect correlation implies that the inverse of matrix $\mathbf{X'X}$ cannot be obtained and therefore more than one solution exists. This problem is known as the existence of exact collinearity or multicollinearity between the independent variables. When the correlation is not exact, it is known as close dependence (*near dependency*) of the independent variables (X). For example, daily coffee consumption and the number of cigarettes smoked daily by the individual might be used to help explain blood pressure levels. When there is strong dependence between coffee consumption and number of cigarettes smoked daily, the estimates of the regression coefficients are not reliable due to the high values obtained in the corresponding variances. However, the effect of this dependence has very little impact on the predictions of the dependent variable. Commonly there is some form of dependence between the independent variables. This dependence becomes a problem when it is too strong. When the dependence is weak, it is often ignored. Chapter 7 introduces the variance inflation factor (VIF), statistic used to detect the presence of multicollinearity. Some of the recommendations to reduce the problem of multicollinearity are (a) in the case of a polynomial regression model, the independent variable must be centralized to reduce multicollinearity between the variables of first order, second order, or higher, and (b) eliminate or combine independent variables (Harrell, 2015).

3.20 Interaction Terms

A special type of linear regression model includes terms formed by the product of predictor variables. For example, the product of the amount of saturated fat in the diet and time spent in moderate-to-vigorous intensity physical activity in the study of blood cholesterol level of adults, which can be defined by the following model:

$$C_i = \beta_0 + \beta_1 F_i + \beta_2 A_i + \beta_3 (\text{FA})_i + e_i \tag{3.20}$$

where C indicates the blood cholesterol levels, F indicates the amount of saturated fat in the diet, A indicates the time spent in moderate-to-vigorous intensity physical activity, and FA indicates the product of the amount of saturated fat in the diet and the time spent in moderate-to-vigorous intensity physical activity (interaction term). The purpose of evaluating the interaction is to determine whether the effect of one predictor variable on the dependent variable varies as a function of a second predictor variable. In this example, the question is whether the effect of the amount of saturated fat in the diet on blood cholesterol levels varies as a function of the time spent in moderate-to-vigorous intensity physical activity. If this term does not have a significant effect, it indicates that the predictor variables are independent of their individual effects on the dependent variable. For example, with the previous model, if we fail to reject H_0: $\beta_3 = 0$, this suggests that the effect of the amount of saturated fat in the diet on blood cholesterol levels does not vary by the time spent in moderate-to-vigorous intensity physical activity. If there is no evidence of a significant interaction term (FA), we fit the model without the interaction term and report the magnitude of the effect of each predictor variable adjusted for the other predictor variable; otherwise, the magnitude of the effect of one predictor variable must be reported at different levels of the other predictor.

3.21 Conclusion

This chapter presents an extension of simple linear regression models, which assesses the contribution of more than one independent variable to explain the dependent variable. Matrix notation is used to facilitate the presentation of least-squares method to estimate the parameters. The chapter also provides an introduction to polynomial regression models, centering of independent variables, and multicollinearity. To complement this chapter, it is recommended to read sections on matrices presented in Draper and Smith (1998), Healy (1992), Kleinbaum et al. (2014), and Rawlings et al. (2001).

Practice Exercise

The following data are concentrations of chlorophyll, phosphorus, and nitrogen taken from several lakes at different times of the day (Manly, 2008):

Lake	Chlorophyll (mg/l)	Phosphorus (mg/l)	Nitrogen (mg/l)
1	95.0	329.0	8
2	39.0	211.0	6
3	27.0	108.0	11
4	12.9	20.7	16
5	34.8	60.2	9
6	14.9	26.3	17
7	157.0	596.0	4
8	5.1	39.0	13
9	10.6	42.0	11
10	96.0	99.0	16
11	7.2	13.1	25
12	130.0	267.0	17
13	4.7	14.9	18
14	138.0	217.0	11
15	24.8	49.3	12
16	50.0	138.0	10
17	12.7	21.1	22
18	7.4	25.0	16
19	8.6	42.0	10
20	94.0	207.0	11
21	3.9	10.5	25
22	5.0	25.0	22
23	129.0	373.0	8
24	86.0	220.0	12
25	64.0	67.0	19

Further details of the data collection can be seen in Smith and Shapiro (1981) and Dominici et al. (1997).

Using matrix algebra, estimate the parameters with 95% confidence intervals of the following linear model:

$$\mu_{\text{chlorophyll}} = \beta_0 + \beta_1 * \text{phosphorus} + \beta_2 * \text{nitrogen}$$

References

Dominici, F., Parmigiani, G., Reckhow, K., and Wolpert, R. (1997) Combining information from related regressions. *J. Agric. Biol. Environ. Stat.*, **2** (3), 313–332.

Draper, N.R. and Smith, H. (1998) *Applied Regression Analysis*, 3rd edition. Hoboken, NJ: John Wiley & Sons, Inc.

Harrell, F.E. (2015) *Regression Modeling Strategies with Applications to Linear Models, Logistic and Ordinal Regression, and Survival Analysis*, 2nd edition. New York, NY: Springer.

Healy, M. (1992) *Matrices for Statistics*. Oxford University Press.

Jewell, N. (2004) *Statistics for Epidemiology*, Boca Raton, FL: Chapman & Hall/ CRC.

Kleinbaum, D.G., Kupper, L.L., Nizam, A., and Rosenberg, E.S. (2014) *Applied Regression Analysis and Other Multivariable Methods*, 5th edition. Boston, MA: Cengage Learning.

Kutner, M.H., Nachtsheim, C., Neter, J., and Li, W. (2004) *Applied Linear Statistical Models*, 5th edition. New York, NY: McGraw-Hill/Irvin.

Manly, B.F.J. (2008) *Statistics for Environmental Science and Management*, 2nd edition. Boca Raton, FL: Chapman &Hall/CRC.

Rawlings, J.O., Pantula, S.G., and Dickey, D.A. (2001) *Applied Regression Analysis: A Research Tool*, 2nd edition. Springer.

Smith, V. and Shapiro, J. (1981) Chlorophyll–phosphorus relations in individual lakes: their importance to lake restoration strategies. *Environ. Sci. Technol.*, **15** (4), 444–451.

4

Evaluation of Partial Tests of Hypotheses in a MLRM

Aim: Upon completing this chapter, the reader should be able to assess partial hypothesis testing in multiple linear regression models.

4.1   Introduction

The selection of a set of independent variables for a multiple linear regression model is a task that involves not only the results observed in a LRM but also the results of previous studies and the experience that the researcher has concerning the problem being investigated. It is important to note that not all the variables that are collected in a study are necessary to adequately explain the variation in the response variable Y. It is desirable to build a regression model containing the "best" subset of variables that affords satisfactory results, according to the objectives of the study. The use of the smallest possible number of variables can reduce costs for future studies.

Rejection of the null hypothesis in Chapter 3 indicated that at least one of the regression coefficients was different from zero. But which one? In some public health studies, it is important to determine whether some subset of independent variables of a MLRM can be equally efficient in their predictions when compared with the model containing all possible predictors. We are particularly interested in assessing the interaction between the exposure and each one of the potentially confounding variables. In this chapter we discuss some strategies to evaluate the elimination of some predictors from the regression model. Other alternatives are provided in the following chapters.

4.2   Specific Objectives

- Define the concept of partial statistical hypothesis in a MLRM.
- Describe the evaluation process of partial statistical hypotheses in a MLRM.

Applications of Regression Models in Epidemiology, First Edition. Erick Suárez,
Cynthia M. Pérez, Roberto Rivera, and Melissa N. Martínez.
© 2017 John Wiley & Sons, Inc. Published 2017 by John Wiley & Sons, Inc.

4.3 Definition of Partial Hypothesis

If the null hypothesis is not rejected in the ANOVA test, then no predictor is useful in explaining the expected value of the response variable, and no further testing is needed. When the null hypothesis is rejected, not all predictors are necessarily essential and we must determine which ones are. One alternative is to conduct hypothesis testing for each coefficient individually. Assuming identically and independently normally distributed regression errors, this is known as a t-test in MLRM. ANOVA essentially tests if the entire model is worthwhile, whereas the t-test assesses if an individual predictor in the model is worthwhile. In simple linear regression, since there is only one predictor, a t-test and an ANOVA lead to equivalent conclusions. But in MLRM they have different interpretations. The problem with the t-test in MLRM is that one predictor is evaluated at a time, conditional on the other predictors in the model, regardless of their significance. Furthermore, the more the predictors in the model, the more the hypothesis tests needed, increasing the chances of incurring in type I and type II errors (Kleinbaum et al., 2014).

ANOVA can be thought as a global F-test procedure. If the null hypothesis is rejected in the global F-test, a partial F-test can be used to determine a subset of predictors that are important. To determine which of the predictors have a nonzero regression coefficient through a partial F-test, the following regression models are used:

i) Complete model

$$E(Y) = \beta_0 + \beta_0 X_1 + \cdots + \beta_m X_m + \beta_{m+1} X_{m+1} + \cdots + \beta_p X_p \qquad (4.1)$$

ii) Incomplete, nested, or reduced model

$$E(Y) = \beta'_0 + \beta'_1 X_1 + \cdots + \beta'_m X_m \qquad (4.2)$$

Note: For simplicity, it is assumed that the first m variables of the complete model form the incomplete model, but of course the incomplete model could be composed differently.

Two models are nested when one model is within the other. For example, $E(Y) = \beta_0 + \beta_1 X_1 + \beta_2 X_2$ is nested within $E(Y) = \beta_0 + \beta_1 X_1 + \beta_2 X_2 + \beta_3 X_3 + \beta_4 X_4$, but $E(Y) = \beta_0 + \beta_1 X_1 + \beta_2 X_2$ is not nested within $E(Y) = \beta_0 + \beta_3 X_3 + \beta_4 X_4$. To determine which of the two models is the best, the following partial hypothesis is established:

$$H_0 : \beta_{m+1} = \beta_{m+2} = \cdots = \beta_p = 0_{|X_1, X_2, \ldots, X_m}$$

This null hypothesis evaluates the $\beta_{m+1}, \beta_{m+2}, \ldots, \beta_p$ coefficients given the presence of $X_1, X_2, \ldots, X_m$ variables in the incomplete model. If this null hypothesis is true, then the incomplete model can produce predictions as good as the complete model.

4.4 Evaluation Process of Partial Hypotheses

To examine the partial hypotheses, it is recommended to carry out the following steps:

i) Calculate the sum of squares of the errors of the complete model, SSE_{com}, with $n - p - 1$ degrees of freedom.

ii) Calculate the sum of squares of the errors of the incomplete model, SSE_{inc}, with $n - m - 1$ degrees of freedom.

iii) Compare the sum of squares for the partial F-statistic, which is defined as follows:

$$F(X_{m+1}, \ldots, X_p | X_1, \ldots, X_m) = \frac{\text{Aditional error sum of squares}}{MSE_{com}}$$

$$= \frac{SSE_{inc} - SSE_{com}/(p - m)}{SSE_{com}/(n - p - 1)} \quad (4.3)$$

This statistic will follow a Fisher F-distribution with $(p - m)$ and $(n - p - 1)$ degrees of freedom if the null hypothesis is true.

iv) Using the Fisher F-distribution with $(p - m)$ and $(n - p - 1)$ degrees of freedom, calculate the p-value.

v) Conclude that there is evidence against H_o if p-value $< \alpha$ (significance level).

4.5 Special Cases

If $m = 0$, then the incomplete model, which consists of the intercept and the test statistic F of ANOVA, evaluates the following hypothesis:

$$H_0 : \beta_1 = \beta_2 = \cdots = \beta_p = 0$$

If $m = p - 1$, then

$$F(X_p | X_1, \ldots, X_{p-1}) = \left(\frac{\beta_p}{se(\beta_p)} \right)^2 = t^2 \quad (4.4)$$

This statistic evaluates the hypothesis $H_0 : \beta_p = 0_{|X_1, X_2, \ldots, X_{p-1}}$. When evaluating only one predictor variable, the partial F equals t^2 and partial F-test conclusions are equivalent to a t-test.

4.6 Examples

Example 1

Assume a MLRM with the following information:

$n = 30$	Total number of subjects
$p = 5$	Total number of independent variables in the complete model
$m = 2$	Total number of independent variables in the incomplete model
$SSE_{com} = 430$	Sum of squares of the errors of the complete model
$SSE_{inc} = 680$	Sum of squares of the errors of the incomplete model

Therefore, the sum of squares for each model will be as follows:

Model	Degrees of freedom	Sum of squares
Complete	24	430
Incomplete	27	680

The null hypothesis evaluates that the regression coefficients associated with the variables X_3, X_4, and X_5 are equal to zero given that X_1 and X_2 are in the model; that is, $H_0 : \beta_3 = \beta_4 = \beta_3 = 0_{|X_1,X_2}$.

The partial F-statistic is defined as

$$\text{partial } F = \frac{(680 - 430)/3}{430/24} = 4.65$$

The Fisher F-distribution percentiles are $F_{(3,24,0.95)} = 3.01$ and $F_{(3,24,0.99)} = 4.72$. Thus, the p-value is between 0.01 and 0.05. This indicates evidence against H_0 at a 5 % significance level; that is, in the incomplete model, at least one of the regression coefficients associated with X_3, X_4, and X_5 is nonzero ($0.01 < p$-value < 0.05). Hence, further analysis is needed to determine which of these three predictors should be kept in the model.

Example 2

Suppose you want to explain the variation in triglycerides levels using waist circumference and age in adults between 21 and 79 years of age (Pérez et al., 2008) in a quadratic model with centralized predictor variables using the data provided in Table 4.1. Therefore, we assume a curvilinear relationship between triglycerides levels and age; we centralize to reduce the effect of multicollinearity given the correlation between age and age squared. The predictor variables in this model are as follows:

waist_c:	Waist circumference in inches centralized with respect to its mean: $$\text{waist}\_c = \text{waist} - \overline{\text{waist}}$$
age_c:	Age centralized with respect to its mean: $$\text{age}\_c = \text{age} - \overline{age}$$
age_c2:	Square of the variable age centralized: $\text{age}\_c2 = \text{age}\_c^2$

The information resulting from using a multiple linear regression with the data of Table 4.1 in STATA is described in Table 4.2.

Therefore, the equation of the MLRM using the results in Table 4.2 is as follows:

$$\hat{\mu}_{\text{Triglycerides}} = 85.68 + 6.98\text{waist}\_c_1 + 0.005\text{age}\_c + 0.023\text{age}\_c_2$$

Table 4.1 Triglycerides levels by waist circumference and age.

Triglycerides level	Waist circumference	Age
28	32.95	38
40	33.0	43
50	33.5	23
61	33.5	42
66	34.5	21
70	37.0	21
79	35.0	44
85	36.85	57
87	36.45	33
89	40.65	63
90	40.5	53
107	43.5	52
109	42.0	23
111	39.4	78
112	40.2	74
119	44.9	40
121	43.5	51
130	44.8	64
149	41.5	22
159	45.0	71

Source: Pérez et al. (2008).

Table 4.2 ANOVA and parameter estimation of a MLRM.

```
ANOVA:
   Source |      SS       df     MS         Number of obs   =      20
---------+---------------------------       F(3, 16)        =   28.79
    Model | 19357.83     3   6452.61        Prob > F        =  0.0000
 Residual |  3585.98    16    224.12        R-squared       =  0.8437
---------+---------------------------       Adj R-squared   =  0.8144
    Total |  22943.8    19  1207.56842      Root MSE        =  14.971
```

Parameter estimation

Triglycerides	Coefficient	Std. error	t	$P > \|t\|$	95% Confidence interval	
waist_c	6.98	0.88	7.94	<0.001	5.12	8.85
age_c	0.01	0.21	0.03	0.98	−.430	0.44
age_c2	0.02	0.01	2.09	0.05	0.00	0.05
_cons	85.68	4.89	17.53	<0.001	75.32	96.04

The ANOVA results in Table 4.2 indicates evidence against the null hypothesis ($H_0 : \beta_1 = \beta_2 = \beta_3 = 0$) at a 5% significance level, that is, at least one of the coefficients of the predictor variables is different from zero (p-value <0.05). Moreover, it has an adjusted $R^2 = 81.4\%$; that is, the model may explain 81.4% of the variability of triglycerides levels when adjusted by the degrees of freedom.

The parameters estimation in Table 4.2 also indicates the significance of each individual predictor variable using t-statistics, as described in Chapter 2. According to these results, age was not significant (p-value >0.10), that is, there is evidence in favor of $H_0 : \beta_2 = 0_{|waist, age^2}$. The quadratic term showed marginal significance (p-value $= 0.05$).

The simultaneous evaluation of the two regression coefficients is performed with the partial tests using the Fisher F-distribution, as described in the previous section. Continuing with the previous model, partial tests to assess simultaneously two coefficients are as follows:

Evaluating the hypothesis $H_0 : \beta_1 = \beta_2 = 0_{|X_3}$

```
F( 2,   16) =   37.51
       Prob > F =    0.0000
```

Evaluating the hypothesis $H_0 : \beta_1 = \beta_3 = 0_{|X_2}$

```
F (   2,     16)  =     35.37
        Prob  >  F  =      0.0000
```

Evaluating the hypothesis $H_0 : \beta_2 = \beta_3 = 0_{|X_1}$

```
F (   2,     16)  =      2.21
        Prob  >  F  =      0.1425
```

The results of the hypothesis tests show that when the variable circumference centralized (X_1) is in the model, the coefficients associated with the variable age centralized (X_2) and the variable age centralized squared (X_3) are not significant (p-value >0.10). However, when X_1 was not present in these partial evaluations, centralized age always showed significant results (p-value <0.05). This may suggest removing age when explaining triglyceride levels in a multiple linear model. It should be noted that when fitting a quadratic model, it is not always best to remove the lower order term, even when nonsignificant. This will depend on the type of quadratic curve deemed appropriate. When drawing a scatterplot of the response versus the predictor, is there approximately a parabolic association? If so, then it is appropriate to remove the lower order term if not significant. Otherwise, when there is no maximum apparent in the scatterplot, it is best to leave the lower order term in.

4.7 Conclusion

This chapter summarizes strategies to evaluate different predictor variables simultaneously through the comparison of two models (complete and incomplete), using the partial F-test. This method helps identify those predictor variables in a MLRM that contribute significantly to explaining the behavior of a continuous random dependent variable. Hypothesis testing can be performed with ANOVA and a t-test as two special cases of these partial tests.

Practice Exercise

Given the information from Example 2 of this chapter to explain the *level of triglycerides* given waist, age, and age^2 using a MLRM,

a) Make the programing in Stata, SAS, R and SPSS to evaluate the hypothesis $H_0 : \beta_2 = \beta_3 = 0_{|waist}$.

References

Kleinbaum, D.G., Kupper, L.L., Nizam, A., and Rosenberg, E.S. (2014) *Applied Regression Analysis and Other Multivariable Methods*, 5th edition. Boston, MA: Cengage Learning.

5

Selection of Variables in a Multiple Linear Regression Model

Aim: Upon completing this chapter, the reader should be able to apply several criteria for choosing predictor variables in a multiple linear regression model.

5.1 Introduction

In Chapter 4, partial F-tests were used to eliminate subsets of predictors that are not useful in modeling the response variable Y. Although type I and type II errors are less likely to be incurred when performing partial F-tests than when using t-tests, the chances of incurring these errors can still be unacceptably high, especially when there is a large number of subsets of predictors to test. Moreover, partial F-test limits our choice of models because it only works when comparing nested models. As a result, a partial F-test procedure may not result in the simplest model. In this chapter, we will apply several other criteria for choosing predictor variables in a multiple linear regression model.

5.2 Specific Objectives

- Describe some criteria used for selecting the best subset of predictors in building a regression model.
- Apply the *stepwise* algorithms in finding the best subset of predictors or explanatory variables.

5.3 Selection of Variables According to the Study Objectives

i) **Descriptive Study:** It is not advisable to remove variables.
ii) **Prediction Study:** The deletion of unnecessary variables provides "economic" benefits. However, caution should be exercised because bias can result in the removal of important variables.

Applications of Regression Models in Epidemiology, First Edition. Erick Suárez,
Cynthia M. Pérez, Roberto Rivera, and Melissa N. Martínez.
© 2017 John Wiley & Sons, Inc. Published 2017 by John Wiley & Sons, Inc.

iii) **Estimation Study:** Be conservative in the elimination of variables. Avoid biases when eliminating important variables from the model.

iv) **Extrapolation Study:** Greater care is needed in the selection of variables for the best explanation of the response variable Y outside the observed values of Xs.

v) **Association studies in epidemiology:** When the interest is to assess the strength of the association between an exposure and disease in an epidemiologic study, caution should be taken to remove the predictors due to the presence of variables that may confound or modify the association of interest. Further details will be provided in Chapter 10.

5.4 Criteria for Selecting the Best Regression Model

There are several criteria that can be used to select the number of independent variables in a regression model. These criteria are based on the principle of parsimony (select the simplest explanation possible that agrees with the evidence), using a minimum of independent variables and attaining a minimum sum of squared errors (SSE). The commonly used criteria are R^2, adjusted R^2, MSE, Mallows's C_p statistic, and two information criteria (Akaike information criterion (AIC) and Bayesian information criterion (BIC)).

5.4.1 Coefficient of Determination, R^2

This criterion selects the model that has the highest R^2 with the lowest number of possible predictors. We choose a model with k predictors if adding another variable does not increase the R^2 substantially. The following are some of the disadvantages with this approach:

- Outliers have great influence on the calculation of R^2.
- A model with few predictors will always have an R^2 less than or equal to a model that includes a larger number of predictors. In other words, the R^2 tends to increase as you increase the number of independent variables.

5.4.2 Adjusted Coefficient of Determination, R_A^2

The limitation with the R^2 criterion is that it does not account for the number of predictors in the model. R_A^2 is based on a modification of the coefficient of determination, which is defined as follows:

$$R_A^2 = 1 - \frac{\text{SSE}/(n - (k + 1))}{\text{SST}/(n - 1)} = 1 - \frac{n - 1}{n - (k + 1)}\left(1 - R^2\right) \tag{5.1}$$

where k is the number of predictors in the multiple linear regression model and n is the number of observations. The best model is one that has a high adjusted

R^2 with minimal independent variables. Unlike the coefficient R^2, the R_A^2 can decrease when you add another independent variable in the model.

5.4.3 Mean Square Error (*MSE*)

Another alternative is to choose the model with the lowest mean squared error, that is,

MSE (Selected model) $\leq$ MSE (Other models)

where $\text{MSE} = \text{SSE}/(n - k - 1)$.

Although SSE will never increase when adding predictors, MSE may increase. This alternative criterion, however, will tend to choose models that are too complex because the penalty for adding unnecessary predictors is not strong enough.

5.4.4 Mallows's C_p

Assuming a multiple linear regression model with p predictors (complete model) is compared with a reduced model (incomplete model) with k predictors ($k < p$), the Mallows's C_p statistic is defined as

$$C_P = \frac{\text{SSE}_{\text{INC}}}{\text{MSE}_{\text{COM}}} + 2(k+1) - n \tag{5.2}$$

where MSE indicates the mean square error of the model with all p predictors and SSE_{inc} indicates the residual sum of squares of the subset model of k predictors.

A model with k predictors is appropriate if $E(C_p) = k + 1$. To choose the value of k, usually a graph is constructed of C_p versus k. The k value most suitable is that closest to the intersection of the graph with the line $C_p = k + 1$.

5.4.5 Akaike Information Criterion

This criterion is based on the Kullback–Leibler distance between the distribution of the response variable under the incomplete model and the distribution of the response variable under the complete model. This measure is defined as

$$\text{AIC}(k) = -2 \ln (\text{SSE}_k) + 2(k+1) \tag{5.3}$$

where SSE_k indicates the residual sum of squares of the model with k predictors.

The appropriate number of variables in the model occurs when AIC reaches its minimum value. This criterion tends to select models with a large number of predictors (West et al., 2015).

5.4.6 Bayesian Information Criterion

In order to avoid selecting models with a large number of predictors, another information criterion is the Schwarz Bayesian Information Criterion, which is defined as follows:

$$BIC(k) = -2 \ln(SSE_k) + (k+1) \times \ln(n) \qquad (5.4)$$

The appropriate number of independent variables in the model is obtained when the BIC reaches its minimum value. This criterion places a higher penalty on models with a larger number of predictors than does the AIC criterion and as a result may choose models with too few predictors (West et al., 2015).

5.4.7 All Possible Models

Conceptually, the only way to ensure the best model for each subset of models from p independent variables is to evaluate all possible models for this set. This is possible when the number of independent variables is small. For example, if 4 predictors are available, then the total number of models is $2^4 - 1 = 15$, distributed as follows:

- Four models with one predictor plus the intercept
- Six models with two predictors plus the intercept
- Four models with three predictors plus the intercept
- One model with four predictors plus the intercept

Table 5.1 presents the results of different linear regression models to explain blood triglyceride levels as a function of waist circumference, hip circumference, high-density lipoprotein cholesterol levels, and age (Pérez et al., 2008).

One alternative for selecting the best model is to determine the subset that meets at least two criteria. In this example it would be the model containing the predictors: *waist, hip,* and *age*. This model has one of the highest R_A^2, one of the lowest AIC and BIC, and a C_p closest to $k+1$.

5.5 *Stepwise* Method in Regression

Stepwise regression sequentially selects (or excludes) the best (or worst) independent variables according to certain pre-established statistical criteria. These criteria do not guarantee to find the best subset of predictors. Moreover, the results obtained by applying different criteria during *stepwise* regression can produce different models. There are three *stepwise* methods or algorithms that are commonly used: *forward selection* (FS), *backward elimination* (BE), and *stepwise selection* (SS), which are described in the following sections.

Table 5.1 Assessment of all possible models for blood triglyceride levels.

k	Variables	R^2	MSE	R_A^2	Mallows's C_p	AIC	BIC
1	waist	0.801	254.17	0.790	−0.4	169.41	171.40
	hip	0.063	1194.35	0.011	57.3	200.36	202.35
	hdl	0.017	1252.41	−0.037	60.9	201.31	203.30
	age	0.153	1080.05	0.106	50.3	198.35	200.34
2	waist, hip	0.803	265.86	0.780	1.4	171.17	174.15
	waist, hdl	0.802	266.82	0.779	1.5	171.24	174.23
	hip, age	0.801	268.26	0.778	1.6	171.35	174.33
	hip, hdl	0.077	1246.27	−0.032	58.3	202.07	205.05
	waist, age	0.153	1143.56	0.053	52.3	200.35	203.33
	hdl, age	0.174	1114.32	0.077	50.6	199.836	202.81
3	waist, hip, hdl	0.805	280.02	0.768	3.3	172.99	176.97
	waist, hip, age	0.807	276.27	0.771	3.1	172.72	176.71
	waist, hdl, age	0.803	282.92	0.766	3.4	173.20	177.18
	hip, hdl, age	0.175	1183.75	0.020	52.6	201.82	205.81
4	waist, hip, hdl, age	0.8083	293.20	0.757	5.0	174.62	179.60

waist indicates waist circumference.
hip indicates hip circumference.
hdl indicates high-density lipoprotein cholesterol.

5.5.1 Forward Selection

This method begins with the selection of the predictor that is most correlated with the response variable. The second predictor to be selected will be the one that meets one of the following requirements:

- The predictor that has the greatest t-statistic, in absolute value, of all predictors not yet included in the model. This is equivalent to choosing the one predictor with the largest partial F (usually greater than 4).
- The predictor that produces the largest increase in the R^2 when added to the model.
- The predictor that has the highest partial correlation (see Chapter 6), in absolute value, with the response variable, given the first predictor is already included in the model.

This process is then continued, adding subsequent predictors until some prespecified condition is reached. For example, one of the criteria used to terminate the selection procedure can be a partial t-test with a certain level of significance, identified by a significance level to enter (SLE) the model. The process ends when the p values of the t-test for variables not yet included in the model are greater than the SLE. Other criteria to terminate the process are as follows:

- The model contains a number of predictors previously set.
- When the significance value of all predictors that were removed from the model is greater than the significance level.

5.5.2 Backward Elimination

In this method, predictors are removed from the complete model. The first predictor to be eliminated is the one that produces the lowest partial F-statistic. This partial F is defined as follows:

$$F_k = \frac{(SSR_k - SSR_{k-1})}{MSE_k} \tag{5.5}$$

where

$\quad SSR_k \quad = $ sum of squares due to regression with k predictors.
$\quad SSR_{k-1} = $ sum of squares due to regression with $k-1$ predictors.
$\quad MSE_k \quad = SSE_k/(n-k-1)$.

The second predictor to be eliminated is the one that produces the next smallest change in F_k from the previous step. Subsequent predictors to be eliminated follow the same process. One of the criteria used to finish eliminating predictors in the model is through partial t-tests with a certain significance level identified by a *significance level to stay* (SLS).

5.5.3 Stepwise Selection

The stepwise regression methods above suffer from the fact that once you have added or removed a predictor, it cannot go out or come in later steps of the algorithm. To overcome this problem, Efroymson (1960) introduces the *Stepwise Selection* algorithm. This method starts the process like *Forward Selection*. From the second predictor onward, each predictor included must meet permanence criteria (the criteria used in the *Backward Elimination*); the predictor with the minimum additional sum of squares is removed. The selection of predictors terminates when all predictors meet the criteria to stay and no variables outside the model meets the entry criteria.

5.6 Limitations of *Stepwise* Methods

At each step of the *Stepwise* methods, one predictor is assessed before moving to the next predictors; so, we cannot select the best model of the subset of models having the same number of predictors. That is, if the selected model has three predictors, we need to analyze all possible models with three predictors and select the best one of them using one or two of the criteria previously discussed (R^2, R^2_{ajus}, MSE, C_P, AIC, or BIC). In general, it is not recommended to use *Stepwise* methods to select the model automatically. Generally, forward selection is preferred when there is a large number of predictors from which some predictors will be kept. Backward elimination is preferred when there are a moderate number of predictors from which some need to be removed. These semiautomatic stepwise regression methods should be used with care, and expertise on the subject matter can be valuable in making the appropriate adjustments. Stepwise regression methods have been criticized with some suggesting that it is best to avoid the techniques (Harrell, 2015). The main criticisms are as follows: R^2 values are biased high, standard errors of the parameter estimates are too small, p-values are too low due to multiple comparisons and are difficult to correct, and influence of multicollinearity on the selection of predictors. The more predictors allowed, the more likely useless predictors will be included (Derksen and Keselman, 1992; Flom and Cassell, 2007). When there are a large number of predictors, another alternative is to use regression methods with restrictions on the value of the regression coefficients. Examples of these methods are ridge regression and least absolute selection and shrinkage operator (known as LASSO) regression methods (Hastie et al., 2011; Hammami et al., 2012).

5.7 Conclusion

In this chapter we present different criteria for selecting the best prediction model when there is more than one predictor. Recommendations are presented to evaluate the need to eliminate predictors in a multiple linear regression model. Finally, we present *Stepwise* methods for selecting the best model and emphasize the limitations of these methods. It is important to keep in mind that in epidemiologic studies, the predictors can be related to the exposure, the confounding variables, and the effect modification variables. As a consequence, the predictors' selection is dependent on the study design, as we will see in Chapters 10–12.

Practice Exercise

The body mass index (BMI) is the content of body fat in relation to height and weight of a person, which is calculated by dividing the weight of each individual in kilograms by the square of height of the individual in meters. The following table shows the BMI, age, total cholesterol, and plasma glucose of 58 adults (Pérez et al, 2008).

BMI	Age	Cholesterol	Glucose	BMI	Age	Cholesterol	Glucose
19.283	21	178	95	31.200	60	216	294
24.542	57	250	98	32.919	28	191	101
24.738	46	176	102	33.117	53	197	100
47.868	47	171	105	25.045	58	196	102
44.220	61	222	101	39.305	53	157	99
29.881	74	156	72	31.295	66	188	209
27.193	22	122	82	35.518	58	186	105
37.844	63	204	115	36.647	75	169	105
25.508	53	164	111	26.586	60	220	100
32.779	40	180	95	35.328	69	189	283
24.401	29	207	79	29.308	68	150	131
33.560	63	135	107	44.638	48	283	99
25.331	24	155	88	36.712	76	176	115
35.518	51	180	302	25.597	41	163	97
30.400	52	240	96	21.063	38	163	100
33.996	25	190	84	24.266	39	153	84
28.956	38	153	107	23.265	65	190	99
26.337	39	207	100	19.418	33	119	78
37.733	58	177	345	27.069	47	185	128
23.635	76	204	95	28.516	37	203	231
22.285	22	156	103	33.816	28	183	93
23.705	69	183	95	32.038	62	242	136
42.891	33	180	91	27.442	35	157	103
25.806	29	157	80	21.668	68	137	93
31.128	34	238	112	30.413	33	216	88
37.398	51	173	95	34.453	49	251	90
34.578	48	259	108	21.042	61	219	91
25.282	28	136	83	26.278	60	178	152
22.269	47	187	90	33.261	40	198	79

a) Determine the best subset of predictors that explain the variability of BMI, using the forward, backward, and stepwise methods.

References

Derksen, S. and Keselman, H.J. (1992) Backward, forward, and stepwise automated subset selection algorithms: frequency of obtaining authentic and noise variables. *Br. J. Math. Stat. Psychol.* **45**, 265–282.

Efroymson, M.A. (1960) Multiple regression analysis. In: Ralston, A. and Wilf, H.S. (eds) *Mathematical Methods for Digital Computers.* New York, NY: John Wiley & Sons, Inc.

Flom, P. and Cassell, D. (2007) *Stopping stepwise: why stepwise and similar selection methods are bad, and what you should use.* NESUG.

Hammami D., Lee, T.S., Ouarda, T., and Lee, J. (2012) Predictor selection for downscaling GCM data with LASSO. *J. Geophys. Res.* **117**, D17116.

Harrell, F.E. (2015) *Regression Modeling Strategies with Applications to Linear Models, Logistic and Ordinal Regression, and Survival Analysis*, 2nd edition. New York, NY: Springer.

Hastie, T., Tibshirani, R., and Friedman, J. (2011) *The Elements of Statistical Learning: Data Mining, Inference, and Prediction*, 2nd edition. New York, NY: Springer Science+Business Media.

Pérez, C., Guzmán, M., Ortiz, A.P., Estrella, M., Valle, Y., Pérez, N., Haddock, L., and Suárez, E. (2008) Prevalence of the metabolic syndrome in San Juan, Puerto Rico. *Ethn. Dis.* **18**, 434–441.

West, B., Welch, K., and Gatecki, A. (2015) *Linear Mixed Models, A Practical Guide Using Statistical Sotware*, 2nd edition. CRC Press.

6

Correlation Analysis

Aim: Upon completing this chapter, the reader should have an understanding of the linear relationship between two or more characteristics of interest in a population.

6.1 Introduction

At times, research on public health problems focuses on the statistical relationship between two or more quantitative random variables (e.g., hemoglobin A1c, blood cholesterol, and insulin levels), without establishing the cause–effect relationship. This occurs particularly in exploratory cross-sectional studies. The goal could be the formulation of a causality hypothesis for future analytic epidemiological studies (Szklo and Nieto, 2007). Often in public health, regression analysis is about analyzing the linear relationship between a response variable and a set of predictors, having in mind a potential cause–effect relationship. With correlation analysis, we measure the degree of the linear relationship among all variables, including between predictors. This chapter describes the different methods of evaluating this linear relationship.

6.2 Specific Objectives

- Describe the different measures of correlation between variables related to MLRM.
- Describe the concepts of partial and semipartial correlations.

6.3 Main Correlation Coefficients Based on SLRM

Assume the following simple linear regression model:

$$Y_i = \beta_0 + \beta_1 X + e_i$$

Applications of Regression Models in Epidemiology, First Edition. Erick Suárez, Cynthia M. Pérez, Roberto Rivera, and Melissa N. Martínez.

where X and Y are quantitative random variables. Based on this model, one can calculate different correlation coefficients, which are described in the following sections.

6.3.1 Pearson Correlation Coefficient ρ

The Pearson correlation coefficient is a parameter that measures the degree and type of linear relationship between two quantitative random variables. This coefficient indicates the degree of linear relationship between X and Y, and takes on values between -1.0 and 1.0. The closer the value of the coefficient to the extreme values of the interval $(-1.0, 1.0)$, the greater the correlation between variables will be. A value close to -1.0 is indicative of a strong inverse linear relationship between the variables, while a value close to 1.0 is indicative of a strong positive linear relationship between the variables. If the coefficient equals zero, it is concluded that there is no linear statistical association between variables. Note that for some nonlinear relationships, such as a parabolic association, which cannot be approximated well by a linear relationship, the correlation coefficient may be zero. That is why graphical displays should also be used when exploring the type of relationship between variables. The parameter is estimated through a sample correlation r. Assuming that X and Y are two quantitative random variables, the sample Pearson correlation coefficient is calculated using the following formula:

$$
\begin{aligned}
r &= \frac{\sum_{i=1}^{n}(x_i - \bar{x})(y_i - \bar{y})}{\sqrt{\sum_{i=1}^{n}(x_i - \bar{x})^2 \sum_{i=1}^{n}(y_i - \bar{y})^2}} \\[2mm]
&= \frac{\sum_{i=1}^{n}(x_i - \bar{x})(y_i - \bar{y})}{\sum_{i=1}^{n}(x_i - \bar{x})^2} \cdot \frac{\sqrt{\sum_{i=1}^{n}(x_i - \bar{x})^2}}{\sqrt{\sum_{i=1}^{n}(y_i - \bar{y})^2}} \\[2mm]
&= \hat{\beta}_i \frac{S_X}{S_Y}
\end{aligned} \tag{6.1}
$$

Table 6.1 shows the possible interpretations for values of the estimated Pearson correlation coefficient.

More precisely, we may interpret an absolute value of the estimated correlation coefficient, $|r|$, between 0.8 and 1 as indicative of strong linear relationship, between 0.3 and 0.79 as indicative of moderate linear relationship, and between 0 and 0.29 as indicative of weak linear relationship (Cohen, 1988).

Table 6.1 Interpretation of the Pearson correlation coefficient.

Value of the coefficient	Interpretation
$0 < r < 1$ and $r \to 1$	Positive linear relationship and strong
$0 < r < 1$ and $r \to 0$	Positive linear relationship and weak
$r = 0$	There is no linear relationship
$-1 < r < 0$ and $r \to -1$	Inverse or negative linear relationship and strong
$-1 < r < 0$ and $r \to 0$	Inverse or negative linear relationship and weak

6.3.2 Relationship Between r and $\hat{\beta}_1$

From the expression (6.1), it can be seen that

$$r = \hat{\beta}_1 \frac{S_X}{S_Y}$$

Therefore,

$$\hat{\beta}_1 = \frac{S_Y}{S_X} r \tag{6.2}$$

Consequently, the estimated simple linear regression equation is

$$\hat{\mu}_{Y|X} = \bar{y} + \hat{\beta}_1 (X - \bar{x}) = \bar{y} + r \left(\frac{S_Y}{S_X} \right) (X - \bar{x}) \tag{6.3}$$

6.4 Major Correlation Coefficients Based on MLRM

The concept of correlation coefficients from the previous section can be extended into a multiple linear regression model. Assume the following model, using the matrix notation:

$$Y_{n \times 1} = X_{n \times (k+1)} \beta_{(k+1) \times 1} + e_{n \times 1} \tag{6.4}$$

Based on this model, various correlation coefficients can be calculated. These are discussed in the following sections.

6.4.1 Pearson Correlation Coefficient of Zero Order

The following matrix shows the correlation between all pairs of variables that make up the regression model, assuming there is a response variable and 3 predictors:

$$
\begin{array}{c}
\begin{array}{cccc} Y & X_1 & X_2 & X_3 \end{array} \\
\begin{array}{c} Y \\ X_1 \\ X_2 \\ X_3 \end{array}
\begin{pmatrix}
1 & r_{Y1} & r_{Y2} & r_{Y3} \\
 & 1 & r_{12} & r_{13} \\
 & & 1 & r_{23} \\
 & & & 1
\end{pmatrix}
\end{array}
$$

where

r_{Yi}: Pearson correlation between Y and X_i

r_{ij}: Pearson correlation between X_i and X_j

Note: The correlation coefficient order means the number of controlled variables to adjust for the correlation index. Zero order indicates a correlation coefficient that is not adjusted by any other variable.

6.4.2 Multiple Correlation Coefficient

The multiple correlation coefficient $R_{Y,\hat{Y}}$ is the correlation coefficient between Y and $\hat{Y}$, that is, between the variable Y and its estimated value based on the regression model. This coefficient is determined by the following formula:

$$
R_{Y,|X_1,...,X_k} = \frac{\sum_{i=1}^{n} (y_i - \bar{y})(y_i - \bar{\hat{y}})}{\sqrt{\sum_{i=1}^{n}(y_i - \bar{y})^2 \sum_{i=1}^{n}(y_i - \bar{\hat{y}})^2}}
\tag{6.5}
$$

where $\bar{\hat{y}}$ is the mean of the regression estimates of the response.

6.5 Partial Correlation Coefficient

The partial correlation coefficient is a measure of the linear relationship between two variables after simultaneously controlling for the effects of one or more independent variables. If the correlation coefficient is calculated controlling for a single variable, it will be a *first-order* partial correlation. If calculated controlling for two variables it will be of second-order partial correlation, and so on. Assuming that the variables of interest are Y and X and the control variables are Z and W, the statistics that can be calculated are the partial correlation coefficients of first and second order.

6.5.1 Partial Correlation Coefficient of the First Order

$$r_{YX|Z} = \frac{r_{YX} - r_{YZ} \cdot r_{XZ}}{\sqrt{\left(1 - r_{YZ}^2\right)\left(1 - r_{XZ}^2\right)}}$$

$$= r_{(Y-\hat{Y})(X-\hat{X})} \quad \text{(Correlation between residuals)}$$

(6.6)

where

$$\hat{Y} = \hat{\beta}_0 + \hat{\beta}_z Z$$
$$\hat{X} = \hat{\beta}_0' + \hat{\beta}_z' Z$$

This coefficient indicates the correlation between Y and X when controlling for the variable Z. This statistic can be calculated from the correlation between the residuals $(Y - \hat{Y})$ and $(X - \hat{X})$, where the fitted values are adjusted for Z.

6.5.2 Partial Correlation Coefficient of the Second Order

$$r_{YX|ZW} = \frac{r_{YX|Z} - r_{YW|Z} \cdot r_{XW|Z}}{\sqrt{\left(1 - r_{YW|Z}^2\right)\left(1 - r_{XW|Z}^2\right)}}$$

$$= r_{(\hat{Y}-Y)(\hat{X}-X)} \quad \text{(Correlation between residuals)}$$

(6.7)

where

$$\hat{Y} = \hat{\beta}_0 + \hat{\beta}_z Z + \hat{\beta}_W W$$
$$\hat{X} = \hat{\beta}_0' + \hat{\beta}_z' Z + \hat{\beta}_W' W$$

This expression indicates the correlation between Y and X when controlling for the variables Z and W. This statistic can be calculated by the correlation between the residuals $(Y - \hat{Y})$ and $(X - \hat{X})$, where the fitted values are adjusted for Z and W.

6.5.3 Semipartial Correlation Coefficient

$$r_{Y(X|Z)} = \frac{r_{YX} - r_{YZ} \cdot r_{XZ}}{\sqrt{1 - r_{XZ}^2}}$$

$$= r_{Y,(X-\hat{X})}$$

(6.8)

$$r_{X(Y|Z)} = \frac{r_{YX} - r_{YZ} \cdot r_{XZ}}{\sqrt{1 - r_{YZ}^2}}$$

$$= r_{X,(Y-\hat{Y})}$$

(6.9)

The term $r_{Y(X|Z)}$ indicates the linear correlation between Y and X, when X is only adjusted for Z. For example, assessing the relationship between cholesterol level (Y) and BMI (X) when controlling for age (Z).

6.6 Significance Tests

To determine if the correlation coefficient is equal to zero ($H_0 : \rho = 0$), you can use the strategy of additional sum of squares (comparison of the sum of squares of the errors between a complete model and one incomplete model) through the Fisher probability F-distribution. For example, to evaluate if $R_{YX_1|X_2,X_3,X_4,X_5}$ is nonzero, the following statistic can be used:

$$F(X_1|X_2,X_3,X_4,X_5) = \frac{\dfrac{\text{SSE}(X_2,X_3,X_4,X_5) - \text{SSE}(X_1,X_2,X_3,X_4,X_5)}{\text{df}_{\text{incomplete}} - \text{df}_{\text{complete}}}}{\dfrac{\text{SSE}(X_1,X_2,X_3,X_4,X_5)}{\text{df}_{\text{complete}}}} \qquad (6.10)$$

where

$\text{df}_{\text{complete}}$:   degrees of freedom of the SSE for the complete model
$\text{df}_{\text{incomplete}}$: degrees of freedom of the SSE for the incomplete model

Based on the probability distribution of F-Fisher, with degrees of freedom ($\text{df}_{\text{incomplete}} - \text{df}_{\text{complete}}$, $\text{df}_{\text{complete}}$), the p-value for the F-statistic is computed.

6.7 Suggested Correlations

To determine certain types of correlation, Kleinbaum et al. (2008) describes different correlations according to the possible relationship among variables X and Y and nuisance variable Z (see Table 6.2).

6.8 Example

Assume a study that is analyzing the following quantitative random variables:

weight indicates the weight (kg)
choles indicates fasting blood cholesterol (mg/dl)
hemog indicates hemoglobin levels (g/dl)
trigl indicates fasting triglyceride levels (mg/dl)
gluco indicates fasting glucose levels (mg/dl)

Table 6.2 Correlations among variables X and Y and nuisance variable Z.

Nuisance relationship	Suggested correlation
X and Y are not affected by Z	r_{XY}
X and Y affected by Z	$r_{YX|Z}$
Only X affected by Z	$r_{Y(X|Z)}$
Only Y affected by Z	$r_{X(Y|Z)}$

The data set available for this study is as follows:

Weight	Choles	Hemog	Trigl	Gluco
64.5	199	12.1	95	92
76.9	245	13.2	153	183
82.5	221	17.5	329	98
77.3	222	10.3	110	86
60.0	161	14.1	91	98
83.1	256	16.3	280	116
94.6	170	16.3	90	89
93.9	165	13.0	78	96
63.0	220	14.0	117	88
64.7	161	12.6	143	154
72.6	189	9.0	149	95
65.9	260	14.4	110	93
75.3	181	14.4	159	83
121.7	116	12.7	73	85
93.3	296	14.5	357	123
64.1	198	12.1	43	91
85.1	140	10.8	50	113
75.2	327	15.3	211	94
60.3	163	13.5	146	93
72.7	159	15.9	71	91
70.0	243	16.0	142	120
64.7	198	13.2	80	89
83.9	162	13.3	95	154
55.6	213	13.2	59	97
47.4	201	12.7	284	102
88.6	233	17.1	265	190
66.8	211	13.7	94	87
89.8	227	13.3	154	92

Table 6.3 Zero-order correlation matrix.

	Choles	Gluco	Hemog	Trigl	Weight
choles	1.00				
gluco	0.15	1.00			
hemog	0.34	0.18	1.00		
trigl	0.58	0.31	0.45	1.00	
weight	−0.13	0.12	0.15	0.09	1.00

Possible correlations that can be obtained from the zero-order correlation matrix (see Table 6.3) are described in Table 6.4.

According to the control variables used to assess the correlation between cholesterol and glucose levels, the calculated value of these correlations changes from positive correlation to small negative correlation when fasting triglyceride levels are part of the control variables.

6.9 Conclusion

This chapter summarizes different correlation statistics that can be evaluated to determine the type of association between continuous random variables. We describe the different types of partial and semipartial correlations that can be explored, when there are more than two variables of interest. Finally, we describe the significance tests to assess the association between two variables when controlling for the presence of other quantitative variables.

Table 6.4 Correlations among variables.

Order	Control variables	Form of correlation	Calculated value
0	–	$r_{choles.gluco}$	0.1495
1	hemog	$r_{choles.gluco|hemog}$	0.0943
1	trigl	$r_{choles.gluco|trigl}$	−0.0352
2	hemog, trigl	$r_{choles.gluco|hemog,trigl}$	−0.0414
2	Only gluco is affected by hemog and trigl	$r_{choles,(gluco|hemog,trigl)}$	−0.0336

Practice Exercise

Using the previous database, determine the correlation between *triglycerides* and *cholesterol* levels when

a) controlling for *hemoglogin* levels

b) controlling for *hemoglobin* and *glucose* levels

c) only *cholesterol* is controlled for *hemoglobin* levels and *weight*.

References

Cohen, J. (1988) *Statistical Power Analysis for the Behavioral Sciences*, 2nd edition. Hillsdale, NJ: Lawrence Erlbaum Associates.

Kleinbaum, D.G., Kupper, L.L., Nizam, A., and Rosenberg, E.S. (2014) *Applied Regression Analysis and Other Multivariable Methods*, 5th edition. Boston, MA: Cengage Learning.

Szklo, M. and Nieto, F.J. (2007) *Epidemiology Beyond the Basics*, 2nd edition. Sudbury, MA: Jones and Bartlett.

7

Strategies for Assessing the Adequacy of the Linear Regression Model

Aim: Upon completing this chapter, the reader should be able to apply different strategies for assessing the basic assumptions of the linear regression models.

7.1   Introduction

This chapter describes some methods to determine whether the assumptions for a linear regression model are met before performing inference. Violation of these assumptions may render inference procedures invalid. When the regression models are constructed, we assume that the relationship of the dependent variable Y to the predictor X is linear, and that the errors are independent and identically distributed as normal random variables with mean 0 and constant variance σ^2. The methods used to assess the model assumptions are called diagnostic procedures and these involve both graphical methods and formal statistical tests.

Violation of the model assumptions can be due to the overall behavior of the observations or due to individual observations. Even when a research protocol is well designed and implemented, it is common to encounter inconsistencies in the data. Some biases may emerge with the collected data because of errors in measurement, errors in data entry, errors in the interview process, errors in the instruments for data collection, errors in the procedures to store the data, errors when the questions are related to the memory skill of the participants, or when the study group is not a random sample of the study population. Procedures to detect problematic observations resulting from these sort of errors will also be described in this chapter.

Applications of Regression Models in Epidemiology, First Edition. Erick Suárez,
Cynthia M. Pérez, Roberto Rivera, and Melissa N. Martínez.
© 2017 John Wiley & Sons, Inc. Published 2017 by John Wiley & Sons, Inc.

7.2 Specific Objectives

- Describe the methods to assess data compliance with the basic assumptions of a linear regression model.
- Identify outliers and influential values in a data set.
- Identify the existence of multicollinearity between the predictors and explanatory variables.
- Describe the procedures for validation of linear regression models.

7.3 Residual Definition

Having defined the most suitable linear regression model, it is necessary to verify compliance with the assumptions necessary for inference. This assessment is conducted primarily through examining the residuals, that is, the differences between observed and fitted values under the model:

$$\hat{e}_i = y_i - \hat{y}_i \tag{7.1}$$

where $\hat{y}_i = \hat{\beta}_0 + \hat{\beta}_1 X_1 + \cdots + \hat{\beta}_p X_p$. The residuals are not the true and unobservable errors, but are rather estimates of the errors based on the observed data.

7.4 Initial Exploration

To describe the methods for assessing the distribution of the residuals, the data described in Table 7.1 will be used (Pérez et al., 2008).

Table 7.1 Example of triglycerides levels (mg/dl) by waist circumference (in.) and age (years).

id	Triglycerides	Waist circumference	Age
1	28	33.0	38
2	40	33.0	43
3	50	33.5	23
4	61	33.5	42
5	66	34.5	21
6	70	37.0	21
7	79	35.0	44
8	85	36.9	57
9	87	36.5	33

Table 7.1 (*Continued*)

id	Triglycerides	Waist circumference	Age
10	89	40.7	63
11	90	40.5	53
12	107	43.5	52
13	109	42.0	23
14	111	39.4	78
15	112	40.2	74
16	119	44.9	40
17	121	43.5	51
18	130	44.8	64
19	149	41.5	22
20	159	45.0	71

The MLRM that is obtained to fit the *level of triglycerides* (*Y*) based on the variables *waist* and *age* is as follows:

$$\hat{Y} = -187.6 + 7.14^*\text{waist} + 0.05^*\text{age}$$

Therefore, the resulting residuals (res $= Y - \hat{Y}$) are as follows:

Y	$\hat{Y}$	res
28	50.21	−22.21
40	50.47	−10.47
50	53.02	−3.02
61	53.99	7.01
66	60.07	5.93
70	77.94	−7.94
79	64.81	14.19
85	79.06	5.94
87	74.98	12.02
89	106.53	−17.53
90	104.59	−14.59
107	125.99	−18.99
109	113.79	−4.79
111	98.00	13.00
112	103.51	8.49

Y	$\hat{Y}$	res
119	135.38	−16.38
121	125.93	−4.93
130	135.89	−5.89
149	110.16	38.84
159	137.67	21.33

Table 7.2 summarizes the residuals. Using a box plot to describe the residuals (Figure 7.1), we observe an asymmetrical pattern around zero due to the fact that the distance between the median and the first quartile (25th percentile) was smaller than the distance between the median and the third quartile (75th percentile). Under normality, a symmetrical pattern in the residuals distribution is expected. In addition, when we display the residuals using a scattergram with the fitted values ($\hat{Y}$) in the x-axis (Figure 7.2), most of the residuals for fitted values greater than 100 are negative; hence, this pattern may suggest a nonuniform distribution pattern in the residuals. This plot can also be used to detect the validity of the linear assumption: A nonlinear pattern in the residuals would indicate that a higher order model is needed. Plotting the residuals against the order of observations is one way of screening for the assumption of independent observations. However, this plot is commonly not too informative. Instead, analysts may rely on study design information and autocorrelation plots to evaluate independence. Several questions should be considered when residual diagnostics are performed: When should the residuals distribution be considered normally distributed? How far should the residuals be from zero? Is there an operational criterion for defining extreme values that affect the fitted values?

Table 7.2 Summary of analysis of residuals.

	Percentiles	Smallest		
1%	−22.2	−22.2		
5%	−20.6	−19.0		
10%	−18.3	−17.5	Obs	20
25%	−12.5	−16.4	Sum of Wgt.	20
50%	−3.9		Mean	0.0005
		Largest	Std. Dev.	15.52
75%	10.3	13.0		
90%	17.8	14.2	Variance	240.85
95%	30.1	21.3	Skewness	0.63
99%	38.8	38.8	Kurtosis	3.04

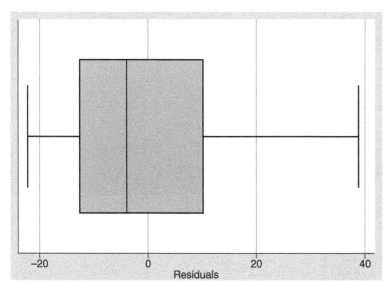

Figure 7.1 Box-and-whisker plot of residuals for waist circumference–blood triglycerides data.

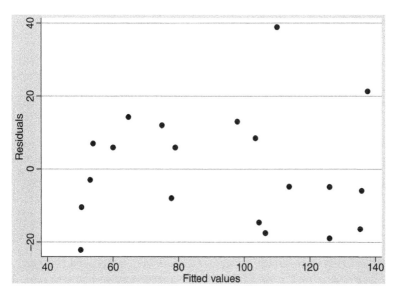

Figure 7.2 Residuals as a function of the fitted values for the waist circumference–blood triglycerides data.

When does a residual indicate an outlier value? Is there some kind of correlation among the residuals? The next sections of this chapter will introduce some of the procedures and statistics for evaluating residuals and operational criteria to determine if the assumptions of the MLRM are met.

7.5 Initial Considerations

In order to assess more closely the assumptions concerning residuals, we should consider the relationship between the fitted values $(\hat{Y})$ and the predictors (X). First notice that

$$\hat{Y} = X\hat{\beta} = X(X'X)^{-1}X'Y = \left(X(X'X)^{-1}X'\right)Y = HY \qquad (7.2)$$

where $H = X(X'X)^{-1}X'$ is defined as the *hat* matrix or projection matrix since it acts as a transformation of Y to $\hat{Y}$. The residuals obtained from the study data depend on Y and X:

$$\hat{e} = Y - \hat{Y} = Y - HY = (I - H)Y \qquad (7.3)$$

As a consequence, the variance of the residuals will be defined as follows:

$$\text{Var}(\hat{e}) = \text{Var}\left(Y - \hat{Y}\right) = \text{Var}(Y - HY) = \text{Var}[(I - H)Y] = (I - H)\sigma^2 \quad (7.4)$$

Given that H is symmetric $(H = H')$ and idempotent $(HH = H)$, each value of the diagonal of the matrix H defines the distance of each observation with respect to its central value $(\overline{X}, \overline{Y})$. This distance, called *leverage*, is identified by h_i and takes values between 0 and 1. The leverage of an observation measures its ability to move the regression model all by itself, by affecting the slope of the model. A point with zero leverage has no effect on the regression model. If a point has leverage equal to 1, the point must be on the regression line. Therefore, different types of residuals are defined to compensate for differences in leverage and other issues in meeting the model assumptions.

7.6 Standardized Residual

This measure is obtained by the ratio of the residual and its standard deviation:

$$\text{Standardized residual} = e'_i = \frac{y_i - \hat{y}_i}{s} \qquad (7.5)$$

where $s = \sqrt{\text{var}(\hat{e})} = \sqrt{\text{MSE}}$.

This residual helps us explore constant variance, one of the most important assumptions in linear regression, and examine observations of high leverage. A violation of the constant variance assumption may impact statistical tests and the length of confidence intervals. To verify compliance with constant variance, it is recommended to graphically represent the standardized residuals and fitted values

$(e_i'$ versus $\hat{y}_i)$, or residuals versus each of the predictors $(e_i'$ versus $X_i)$. With enough observations, the standardized residuals e_i' will have a distribution similar to a random variable with Student's t-distribution with $n - k - 1$ degrees of freedom, with the exception that the numerator and denominator are not independent and should follow approximately a standard normal distribution (Rawlings et al., 2001). However, the distribution of standardized residuals is useful for establishing an operational criterion for the range of the most likely values of the e_i'.

Another tool for exploring potential trends of the residuals is the LOWESS method or *locally weighted smoother* (Figure 7.3). This method estimates the value of Y_0 at X_0 using the *weighted least-squares fit* in a small *bandwidth* around X_0 (Hastie et al., 2011). The weighted factor is defined with the following *tricube* function:

$$W(u) = \left(1 - u^3\right)^3$$

where

$$u = \frac{|X_0 - X_i|}{\Delta}$$

Here Δ indicates the largest distance between X_0 and the rest of the points within the bandwidth.

In Figure 7.3, the residuals behave randomly around zero with a small trend toward positive residuals for small fitted values and negative residuals for large

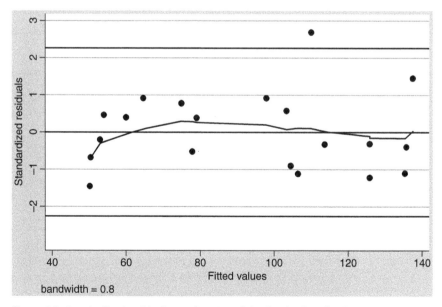

Figure 7.3 Standardized residuals as a function of the fitted values for the waist circumference–blood triglycerides data with LOWESS smoothing.

fitted values. One of the residuals deviates more than 2 units from zero. Further on, criteria are described to formally determine if this distance from zero is significant.

7.7 Jackknife Residuals (R-Student Residuals)

To detect outliers, an alternative is to standardize each residual based on an estimate of the standard deviation that is independent of the corresponding residual. This can be achieved by estimating the MSE obtained from a model that omits observation i; a model with $n - 1$ observations. The notation of this estimate is $s^2_{(-i)}$, where the index $-i$ indicates that the observation i has been removed to estimate σ^2. The result of this estimation leads to the computation of a Jackknife residual:

$$e_{(-i)} = \frac{e_i}{\sqrt{s^2_{(-i)}(1 - h_i)}} = e'_i * \sqrt{\frac{(n - k - 1) - 1}{(n - k - 1) - (e'_i)^2}} \tag{7.6}$$

Jackknife residuals have a mean near 0 and a variance that is slightly greater than 1 (Figure 7.4). According to the central limit theorem, for large enough data it is

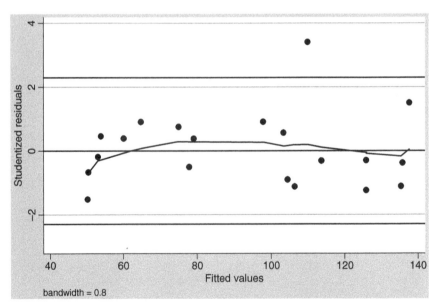

Figure 7.4 Jacknife residuals as a function of the fitted values for the waist circumference–blood triglycerides data with LOWESS smoothing.

expected that these residuals follow approximately a standard normal distribution, if the data meet the condition of normality.

7.8 Normality of the Errors

Statistical t- and F-tests are used to determine statistical significance of predictors if the assumption of normality of the errors is met. To evaluate this assumption, normality graphs can be used. This graph consists of a plane where the x-axis contains the expected ordered values of the standard normal z and the y-axis represents the residuals sorted by magnitude (lowest to highest). This type of graph is called *quantile–quantile* plot for the residuals. If the residuals come from a normal distribution, the plot should resemble a straight line. In Figure 7.5 the normality graph for standardized residuals is displayed from our example. This figure shows that the residuals of the triglycerides follow a linear trend with the exception of the observation at the upper end; therefore, we can say that the residuals are approximately normally distributed.

Another way to evaluate the normality of a data set is through the Shapiro–Wilk test. The test statistic W' is defined as the square of the correlation between $\hat{e}_i$ and $z_{(i)}$:

$$W' = \frac{\left(\sum_i \left(\hat{e}_i - \bar{\hat{e}}\right) z_{(i)}\right)^2}{\sum_i \left(\hat{e}_i - \bar{\hat{e}}\right)^2 \sum_i z_{(i)}^2} \tag{7.7}$$

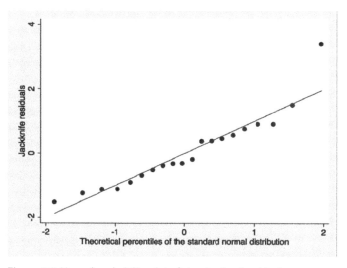

Figure 7.5 Normal probability plot of standardized residuals.

Table 7.3 Shapiro–Wilk W test for normal data.

Variable	Obs	W	V	z	Prob z
residstd	20	0.949	1.204	0.375	0.354

where

$\hat{e}_i =$ value of the ith residual

$\bar{\hat{e}} =$ average of the residuals

$z_{(i)} =$ percentile value under the standard normal distribution corresponding to the area p_i: $z_{(i)} = \Phi^{-1}(p_i)$, where

$$p_i = \frac{R_i - (3/8)}{n + (1/4)}$$

R_i is the rank of the ith residual after sorting the residuals in ascending order.

W' can be calculated with any residual. The condition of normality is accepted when W' is a high number, that is, when there is a correlation between $\hat{e}_i$ and $z_{(i)}$. The test results with the STATA command *swilk* for previous data are shown in Table 7.3. The results in Table 7.3 indicate that H_0 should not be rejected (*p*-value >0.05), and that the residuals are thus normally distributed.

7.9 Correlation of Errors

To assess the assumption of independence of the errors (and hence of the observations), we plot the residuals versus the order of the observations. Dependence of the errors' means that knowing say the first error can help us "predict" what the next error will be, or help us predict errors at fixed leaps forward. Dependence usually occurs with time series data (data indexed in time). It may also occur in a misspecified model (building a linear model for a nonlinear association), or due to other aspects of how the data were gathered.

Unfortunately, in practice, it is hard to determine from the plot of the residuals versus the order of the errors whether the independence assumption has been violated. The Durbin–Watson test provides a way to analyze the correlation between residuals. This test measures the degree of correlation between consecutive residuals by calculating the following statistic:

$$d = \frac{\sum_{i=2}^{n} (\hat{e}_i - \hat{e}_{i-1})^2}{\sum_{i=1}^{n} \hat{e}_1^2} \approx 2(1 - \hat{\rho}) \tag{7.8}$$

where $\hat{\rho}$ is the serial correlation coefficient between two consecutive residuals, $\hat{\rho}(e_i, e_{i-1})$. The Durbin–Watson statistic d decreases as the serial correlation increases.

Table 7.4 Durbin–Watson test with normal *p*-value.

dw	Prob < dw	Prob > dw
1.219	0.0208	0.979

STATA commands:
reg trigl waist age
ttsee id
dwe
*dwe command should be downloaded previously and run
with the command tsset.

The *d* statistic can be used to evaluate the correlation between the residuals and to test the null hypothesis $H_0 : \rho = 0$ versus $H_a : \rho > 0$. The significance level of the *d* statistic can be determined using the *dwe* command in STATA, which generates two *p*-values according to the alternative hypothesis (see Table 7.4).

For the example above, we use the second *p*-value (Prob > dw) when the alternative hypothesis indicates that the serial correlation coefficient is greater than zero; so, in this case the results indicate that there is no evidence of serial correlation between consecutive residuals (*p*-value > 0.05).

7.10 Criteria for Detecting *Outliers, Leverage, and Influential Points*

Outliers in a data set are those observations whose values behave differently from the rest of the observations, with residuals being much larger or smaller. Outliers can increase the variance of regression coefficients and hence make inference less reliable. Leverage points can be thought of as outlying predictor values, and may represent a combination of unusual values of several predictors. High leverage points can give too much weight to some values of *Y* when fitting the regression model, and this can influence coefficient estimates. Influential points are those whose removal and refitting of the model results in large changes in coefficient estimates. An influential point may either be an outlier or have a large leverage, or both, but it will have at least one of those properties.

In linear regression analysis, there are two procedures for determining the presence of outliers. The first is to observe the graph of residuals versus the fitted values and the graph of normality. The second method is to compute a numerical expression to determine whether or not observations are atypical. These numerical methods are described in the sections below.

On a graph of standardized residuals (Figure 7.3), if points are above 2 or below −2, then these points may be *outliers*. In a graph of normality, if the points are far from the straight line, it is also possible that they are outliers (Figure 7.5).

7.11 Leverage Values

For observation y_i in a model with p predictors and sample of size n, it is advisable to evaluate this observation when $h_i > (2(p + 1))/n$, since it may have high leverage in the model (Rawlings et al., 2001). Using the information of the previous example, we obtain the following limit:

$$\frac{2(p + 1)}{n} = \frac{2(2 + 1)}{20} = 0.3$$

The distribution of the *leverage* values according to the id (sequential number) of the subject is given in Figure 7.6.

According to this graph, the *leverage* values of the observations are within the predetermined range, less than 0.3. Therefore, no observation appears to be an outlier.

7.12 Cook's Distance

This statistic determines the magnitude of the change in regression coefficients attributable to the elimination of the ith observation. Therefore, Cook's distance

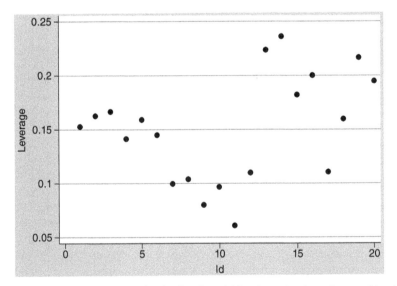

Figure 7.6 Leverage values for the fitted model for the waist circumference–blood triglycerides data by subject's id.

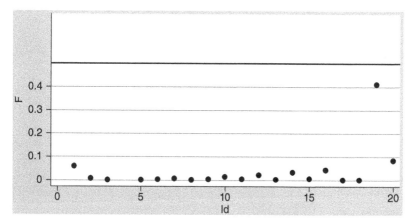

Figure 7.7 Cumulative area of Cook's distance for the waist circumference–blood triglycerides data.

measures the influence of the ith observation on coefficient estimates. The formula is given by

$$D_i = \frac{\left(\hat{\beta}_{(-i)} - \hat{\beta}\right)'(X'X)\left(\hat{\beta}_{(-i)} - \hat{\beta}\right)}{(p+1)s^2} = \frac{\hat{e}_i^2 h_i}{(p+1)s^2(1-h_i)^2} \tag{7.9}$$

If removing the ith observation does not affect the estimation of the β parameters, then the D_i statistic follows a Fisher F-distribution with $(p+1)$ and $(n-p-1)$ degrees of freedom. If the cumulative area to D_i, under the Fisher F-distribution, is greater than 50%, the distance $(\hat{\beta}_{(-i)} - \hat{\beta})$ should be considered large, which implies that the observation i has a substantial effect on the model fit. The D_i statistics corresponding to the observations in our example are displayed in Figure 7.7.

None of the values of the D statistic in Figure 7.7 is greater than 50% (denoted by the horizontal line). Therefore, we cannot say that there are influential values.

7.13 COV RATIO

Another measure of influence is the COV ratio. This measure indicates the change in the accuracy of the estimates of the parameters if an observation is removed. The formula of the COV ratio is presented below:

$$\text{COVRATIO}_i = \frac{\det\left[s_{(-i)}^2\left(X'_{(-i)}X_{(-i)}\right)^{-1}\right]}{\det\left[s^2(X'X)^{-1}\right]} \tag{7.10}$$

where

$$s^2 = \text{estimated variance}$$
$$s^2_{(-i)} = \text{variance estimated without the } i\text{th observation}$$
$$\det[A] = \text{determinant of the matrix A}$$
$$X_{(-i)} = \text{matrix } X \text{ without the } i\text{th observation}$$
$$X'_{(-i)} = \text{transpose of the matrix } X_{(-i)}$$

When all observations have equal influence on the variance of the coefficients, the COV ratio should be close to 1. When the value of the COVRATIO for the ith observation is outside the bounds set by $1 \pm (3(p+1))/n$, where p is the number of predictor variables, it is necessary to evaluate the corresponding observation. The limits for the current data set being analyzed are the following:

$$1 - \frac{3(p+1)}{n} = 1 - \frac{3(2+1)}{20} = 0.55$$

$$1 + \frac{3(p+1)}{n} = 1 + \frac{3(2+1)}{20} = 1.45$$

That is, the ith observation is influential if its COVRATIO is outside the interval $(0.55, 1.45)$.

7.14 DFBETAS

The DFBETAS is a standardized measure of the impact of observations on the estimated regression coefficients, and is calculated as follows:

$$\text{DFBETAS}_{j(i)} = \frac{\hat{\beta}_j - \hat{\beta}_{j(-i)}}{s_i \sqrt{c_j}} \tag{7.11}$$

where

$$\hat{\beta}_j = \text{estimated coefficient for the } j\text{th variable}$$
$$\hat{\beta}_{j(-i)} = \text{estimated coefficient for the } j\text{th variable without}$$
$$\text{the } i\text{th observation}$$
$$s_i = \text{estimated standard error}$$
$$c_j = j\text{th element of the diagonal of } (X'X)^{-1}$$

Absolute values of DFBETAS greater than $2/\sqrt{n}$ indicate points of influence on $\hat{\beta}_j$. So, in our example, DFBETAS with values larger than 0.45 will have an impact on the estimated regression coefficients.

7.15 DFFITS

DFFITS is a measure that evaluates the standardized difference between the fitted model that eliminates the ith observation and the fitted model containing all the observations. The formula for this measure is as follows:

$$\text{DFFITS}_i = \frac{\hat{y}_i - \hat{y}_{i(-i)}}{s_{(-i)}\sqrt{h_i}}$$

(7.12)

where

$\hat{y}_i$ = estimate of the ith observation in the model with all observations

$\hat{y}_{i(-i)}$ = estimate of the ith observation in the model without this observation

$s_{(-i)}$ = standard error estimated without the ith observation

h_i = ith element of the diagonal of the matrix H

A criterion for determining whether an observation affects the fitted values is when the absolute value of DFFITS exceeds $2^*\sqrt{(p+1)/n}$, where p is the number of predictor variables (Rawlings et al., 2001). In our example, DFFITS with values larger than 0.77 will have an impact on the fitted values.

7.16 Summary of the Results

Examples of the values of *leverages*, Cook's distance, COVRATIO, DFBETAS, and DFFITS with the data set in the previous example are described in Table 7.5. The information provided in this table shows that some caution is needed for observations in bold which were outside of the expected ranges for the COVRATIO, DFBETAS, or DFFITS statistics. It is recommended to review the original data in case the data were incorrectly stored, read, or classified, or if the data were from another population. If an issue is identified, a decision should be taken to remove these observations as the last resource or to report this limitation of the study. Another option is to use a robust regression model to explore whether these data points are data entry errors, or from a different population, and therefore there would be no compelling reason to exclude these data points from the analysis. Robust regression might be a good strategy since it is a compromise between excluding these points entirely from the analysis and including all the data points and treating all of them equally in ordinary least-squares (OLS) regression. The idea of robust regression is to weigh observations differently based on how well behaved these observations are. Roughly speaking, it is a form of weighted least-squares regression. The following section will explain weighted regression models.

7.17 Multicollinearity

In studies using regression analysis, the goal is to explore the dependence between the response variable Y and the predictors X_i. However, if there is

Table 7.5 Summary of regression diagnostics.

id	lev	dcook	covratio	dfwaist	dfage	dffits
1	0.152	0.130	0.941	**0.507**	−0.065	−0.648
2	0.162	0.031	1.313	0.250	−0.080	−0.302
3	0.166	0.003	1.428	0.041	0.038	−0.088
4	0.141	0.012	1.345	−0.145	0.040	0.183
5	0.159	0.010	1.387	−0.051	−0.096	0.167
6	0.145	0.015	1.336	−0.014	0.160	−0.211
7	0.100	0.031	1.146	−0.212	0.069	0.302
8	0.104	0.006	1.304	−0.072	0.080	0.127
9	0.080	0.017	1.174	−0.057	−0.089	0.222
10	0.097	0.045	1.053	−0.006	−0.232	−0.371
11	0.061	0.018	1.097	−0.047	−0.059	−0.232
12	0.110	0.062	1.020	−0.306	0.031	−0.438
13	0.223	0.011	1.515	−0.112	0.140	−0.173
14	0.236	0.085	1.353	−0.160	**0.445**	0.501
15	0.182	0.024	1.383	−0.053	0.221	0.264
16	0.200	0.104	1.193	−0.479	0.278	−0.563
17	0.111	0.004	1.325	−0.078	0.012	−0.109
18	0.160	0.010	1.389	−0.100	−0.045	−0.166
19	0.217	0.659	**0.297**	**1.089**	−1.482	**1.793**
20	0.195	0.169	1.003	0.355	0.334	0.738

dependence among the predictors, regression coefficients of the predictors X_i may be indeterminate or have very large standard errors. This implies that there are redundancies among the predictors; essentially the same information is being provided in more than one way. If the dependence among the predictor variables is very strong, *multicollinearity* is said to exist. Some criteria used to detect multicollinearity are the following:

- A model with elevated R^2 but nonsignificant t-statistics.
- A regression coefficient with a sign opposite to that expected.
- Deletion of a row or a column of the matrix X produces large changes in the adjusted model.
- The correlation coefficient between pairs of explanatory variables is very high (e.g., $r_{\beta_i,\beta_j} \geq 0.8$).

Multicollinearity can also be detected using what is known as the variance inflation factor or VIF_j. For each explanatory variable X_j, the VIF is defined by the following formula:

$$VIF_j = \frac{1}{1 - R_j^2} \qquad (7.13)$$

where R_j^2 indicates the coefficient of determination under the model

$$X_j = \beta_0 + \beta_1 X_1 + \cdots + \beta_k X_k + e_i.$$

In this model, one of the independent or predictor variables is explained by the other predictor variables, and the model contains $k - 1$ variables. The variable X_j is dependent on other predictors if its VIF_j is greater than 10.

When we analyzed the multicollinearity of the data set shown at the beginning of the chapter, the criteria of the variance inflation factor are described in Table 7.6. Neither of the VIF in Table 7.6 exceed 10 and it is concluded that there are no problems of collinearity between the predictor variables.

Another approach is to use the *condition number* of the matrix $X'X$ defined by

$$K(x) = \sqrt{\frac{\lambda_{max}}{\lambda_{min}}} \qquad (7.14)$$

where $\lambda_{max}, \lambda_{min}$ denote the extreme *eigenvalues* of the matrix $X'X$.

The eigenvalues $\lambda_1, \lambda_2, \ldots, \lambda_n$ of a matrix A_{nxn} represent the roots that provide solutions to the equation:

$$|A - \lambda I| = 0$$

The larger the quotient $K(x)$, the greater the degree of multicollinearity. An operational criterion that indicates multicollinearity problems is $K > 30$. Some of the recommendations to reduce multicollinearity problems are (i) center the values of the predictor variables, $X_i - \overline{X}$, (ii) combine predictor variables, or (iii) in case of two highly correlated variables ($r > 0.9$) use only one in the model.

Table 7.6 Variance inflation factor.

Variables	VIF	1/VIF
Waist	1.2	0.831
Age	1.2	0.831
Mean VIF	1.2	

7.18 Transformation of Variables

Several strategies were described to evaluate whether the assumptions are met for an OLS regression model. When problems are detected, transformation of the variables is an option. The three basic reasons for transforming variables in regression are as follows: (i) to simplify relationships, (ii) to fix nonnormality in the dependent variable, and (iii) to correct heterogeneous variances of the errors.

Transformation to simplify relationships is to empirically determine mathematical forms of the dependent and independent variables that allow the observed relationship to be represented in a simpler form, preferably a straight line (Draper and Smith, 1998). Transformation options include those in the power family $X^* = X^k$ or $Y^* = Y^k$. The common powers considered are $K = -1$, $-1/2$, 0, 1/2, 1, 2 where the power transformation $k = 0$ is to be interpreted as the logarithmic transformation.

The appropriate transformation to stabilize variance depends on the relationship between the variance and the mean of the dependent variable (Y). When Y follows a Poisson distribution, the recommended variance-stabilizing transformation is $\sqrt{Y}$ or $1/2\{Y^{1/2} + (Y + 1)^{1/2}\}$. When Y follows a binomial distribution, the recommended variance stabilizing transformation is $\sin^{-1}\left(\sqrt{Y}\right)$ or

$$\frac{1}{2}\left[\sin^{-1}\left\{\frac{n_i Y_i}{n_i + 1}\right\}^{1/2} + \sin^{-1}\left\{\frac{n_i Y_i + 1}{n_i + 1}\right\}^{1/2}\right]$$

where n_i is the sample size under different conditions.

Transformation to improve normality has been given lower priority than the other two types of transformations because normality is not required for the OLS estimation, rather only for inference. Fortunately, transformation to stabilize variance often improves normality. The $\ln[Y/(1 - Y)]$ and $\sin^{-1}(\sqrt{Y})$ transformations used to stabilize variance and obtain linear relationships also make the distribution of Y more bell-shaped. Likewise, the power family of transformations is also useful for increasing symmetry of the distribution (Rawlings et al., 2001).

7.19 Conclusion

Different criteria to validate the assumptions of a linear regression model for a given data set are presented in this chapter. We start by showing the various transformations that can be carried out with residuals for evaluating their distribution. Statistics are also discussed to evaluate constant variance, normality, and correlations between residuals. It also describes the statistic known as Cook's distance to formally evaluate the extreme values in the residuals. One of the typical methods used to carry out these validations is to eliminate an observation and compare the result in both residuals and the estimation of parameters. Finally, we show the effect of the correlation or multicollinearity between the predictors, detection, and correction strategies.

Practice Exercise

Some studies have shown a positive relationship between the amount of ozone in the air and increased mortality from circulatory and respiratory diseases. Using the following data, fit a regression model for predicting ozone levels as a function of the amount of solar radiation, temperature, and wind speed.

Ozone	Radiation	Temperature	Wind speed	Ozone	Radiation	Temperature	Wind speed
2.76	230	75	10.9	4.31	294	86	8.6
2.76	259	76	15.5	4.86	223	79	5.7
4.00	253	83	7.4	3.33	279	76	7.4
4.79	207	90	8.0	2.84	14	71	9.2
3.11	322	68	11.5	4.90	225	94	2.3
4.00	175	83	4.6	3.68	275	86	7.4
2.52	7	74	6.9	3.39	83	81	6.9
3.94	285	84	6.3	3.56	212	79	9.7
3.42	314	83	10.9	2.52	77	82	7.4
4.27	197	92	5.1	2.35	27	76	10.3
3.39	323	87	11.5	3.33	284	72	20.7
3.11	193	70	6.9	2.62	131	76	8.0
2.35	238	64	12.6	4.25	276	88	5.1
4.50	189	93	4.6	3.45	190	67	7.4
3.61	95	87	7.4	4.14	291	90	13.8

a) Graph the jackknife residuals distribution using a normal quantile plot.

b) Graph the leverage values against the observation's identification number (id), indicating the suggested limit for influential values.

c) Graph the statistic DFFITS, indicating the suggested limit for influential values.

References

Draper, N.R. and Smith, H. (1998) *Applied Regression Analysis*, 3rd edition. Hoboken, NJ: John Wiley & Sons, Inc.

Hastie, T., Tibshirani, R., and Friedman, J. (2011) *The Elements of Statistical Learning: Data Mining, Inference, and Prediction*, 2nd edition. New York, NY: Springer Science+Business Media.

Pérez, C., Guzmán, M., Ortiz, A.P., Estrella, M., Valle, Y., Pérez, N., Haddock, L., and Suárez, E. (2008) Prevalence of the metabolic syndrome in San Juan, Puerto Rico. *Ethn. Dis.*, **18**, 434–441.

Rawlings, J.O., Pantula, S.G., and Dickey, D.A. (2001) *Applied Regression Analysis: A Research Tool*, 2nd edition. Springer.

8

Weighted Least-Squares Linear Regression

Aim: Upon completing this chapter, the reader should be able to include a weighting factor in the linear regression model.

8.1 Introduction

Homogeneity of variance (homoscedasticity) is an assumption required to justify the use of t- and F-tests when performing inference on the coefficients of a linear regression model. This assumption is also required to construct confidence intervals for coefficients or prediction intervals associated with the response variable. As stated in Chapter 7, when the assumption of constant variance does not hold, the ordinary least squares estimates of the regression coefficients tend to have variances that are too high. This chapter discusses the use of *weighted least squares* (WLS) as a strategy to correct the lack of homoscedasticity in the errors.

8.2 Specific Objectives

- Describe the WLS regression models.
- Apply the matrix notation of the WLS model.

8.3 Regression Model with Transformation into the Original Scale of Y

Suppose a multiple linear regression model, $Y = X\beta + e$, where is a model where the error variance is not constant and the covariances are zero, that is,

$$\text{Var}(e_i) = \text{Var}(y_i) = a_i^2 \sigma^2 = \text{Diag}(V)\sigma^2 \qquad (8.1)$$

Applications of Regression Models in Epidemiology, First Edition. Erick Suárez, Cynthia M. Pérez, Roberto Rivera, and Melissa N. Martínez.
© 2017 John Wiley & Sons, Inc. Published 2017 by John Wiley & Sons, Inc.

where $\text{Diag}(V) = (a_1^2, a_2^2, \ldots, a_n^2)$ is the diagonal of the matrix V, defined by

$$V = \begin{pmatrix} a_1^2 & 0 & \cdots & 0 \\ 0 & a_2^2 & \cdots & 0 \\ \vdots & \vdots & \ddots & \vdots \\ 0 & 0 & \cdots & a_n^2 \end{pmatrix} \tag{8.2}$$

given $\text{Cov}(e_i, e_j) = 0$, when $i \neq j$.

The variance of a random variable (say, Y) is affected when it is multiplied by a constant c, as follows:

$$\text{Var}(cY) = c^2 \text{Var}(Y)$$

Therefore, if the constant c is proportional to the reciprocal of the standard deviation of Y, that is,

$$c = \frac{k}{\sqrt{\text{Var}(Y)}}$$

we can establish the following relationship:

$$\text{Var}(cY) = \left(\frac{k}{\sqrt{\text{Var}(Y)}}\right)^2 \text{Var}(Y) = k^2 \tag{8.3}$$

where cY is a transformation of the random variable Y (*rescaled variable*). Under this transformation, the variance is constant; therefore, we can apply the method of *ordinary least squares* (OLS) to estimate the coefficients of the regression model.

This is the principle followed in the method of WLS. The variable Y is transformed so that $V = I$. For example, given the following linear regression model,

$$y_i = \beta_0 + \beta_1 x_{1i} + \cdots + \beta_p x_{pi} + e_i \tag{8.4}$$

or

$$y_i = \beta_0 x_{0i} + \beta_1 x_{1i} + \cdots + \beta_p x_{pi} + e_i \tag{8.5}$$

where $x_{0i} = 1$. Suppose that the residuals are independent with variance $\text{Var}(e_i) = a_i^2 \sigma^2$. If we transform Y using the inverse of the corresponding a_i, we have the following model:

$$\frac{y_i}{a_i} = \beta_0 \frac{x_{0i}}{a_i} + \beta_1 \frac{x_{1i}}{a_i} + \cdots + \beta_p \frac{x_{pi}}{a_i} + \frac{e_i}{a_i} \tag{8.6}$$

The above model can also be expressed as follows:

$$y_i^* = \beta_0 x_{0i}^* + \beta_1 x_{1i}^* + \cdots + \beta_p x_{pi}^* + e_i^* \tag{8.7}$$

In this model the variance of e_i^* turns out to be the constant σ^2. Therefore, if we use the OLS method, we can obtain the best linear *unbiased estimators* for the regression coefficients $\left(\hat{\beta}_0, \hat{\beta}_1, \ldots, \hat{\beta}_p\right)$.

8.4 Matrix Notation of the Weighted Linear Regression Model

Let $V^{1/2}$ be the diagonal matrix consisting of the square roots of the diagonal elements of V. Therefore, $V^{1/2}V^{1/2} = V$. Let W be the transforming matrix of Y to obtain a constant variance defined by

$$W = \left(V^{1/2}\right)^{-1}$$

$$W = \begin{pmatrix} 1/a_1 & 0 & \cdots & 0 \\ 0 & 1/a_2 & \cdots & 0 \\ \vdots & \vdots & \ddots & \vdots \\ 0 & 0 & \cdots & 1/a_n \end{pmatrix} \tag{8.8}$$

where a_i are constants that indicate the proportional difference of the variances of the residuals. Note that $WW = V^{-1}$. By multiplying both sides of the model Y by the matrix W, we obtain

$$WY = WX\beta + We$$

or

$$Y^* = X^*\beta + e^* \tag{8.9}$$

Therefore, the variance of ϵ^* is constant given the definition of W:

$$\begin{aligned} \mathrm{Var}(e^*) &= \mathrm{Var}(We) \\ &= W\,\mathrm{Var}(e)W' \\ &= WVW\sigma^2 \\ &= I\sigma^2 \end{aligned}$$

given that $WVW = \left(V^{1/2}\right)^{-1}V^{1/2}V^{1/2}\left(V^{1/2}\right)^{-1} = I$.

Now that the variances are constant, it is possible to apply the OLS method to estimate the regression coefficient (β) of Y^* given X^*. Therefore, the WLS estimation of the β coefficients is given by

$$\hat{\beta}_W = (X^{*\prime}X^*)^{-1}X^{*\prime}Y^* = (X'W'WX)^{-1}(X'W'WY) = (X'V^{-1}X)^{-1}(X'V^{-1}Y) \tag{8.10}$$

The variance of $\hat{\beta}_W$ is

$$\mathrm{Var}(\hat{\beta}_W) = (X^{*\prime}X^*)^{-1}\sigma^2 = (X'V^{-1}X)^{-1}\sigma^2$$

The WLS method is equivalent to the OLS method applied to the transformed variable Y^*. Model analysis focuses on the transformed variable $\hat{Y}^* = X^*\hat{\beta}_W$ estimates with the following changes:

i) Estimation of the variable Y on the original scale is $\hat{Y}_W = W^{-1}\hat{Y}^* = X\hat{\beta}_W$

ii) The corresponding variances of $\hat{Y}^*$ and $\hat{Y}_W$ are

$$\mathrm{Var}\left(\hat{Y}^*\right) = X^*\left(X'V^{-1}X\right)^{-1}X^{*'}\sigma^2 \tag{8.11}$$

$$\mathrm{Var}\left(\hat{Y}_W\right) = X\left(X'V^{-1}X\right)^{-1}X'\sigma^2 \tag{8.12}$$

iii) The observed residuals are as follows:
- Transformed variable:

$$e^* = Y^* - \hat{Y}^* \tag{8.13}$$

- Variable on the original scale:

$$e = Y - \hat{Y}_W \tag{8.14}$$

iv) The corresponding variances of the residuals are as follows:
- Transformed variable:

$$\mathrm{Var}(e^*) = \left(I - X^*\left(X'V^{-1}X\right)^{-1}X^{*'}\right)\sigma^2 \tag{8.15}$$

- Variable on the original scale:

$$\mathrm{Var}(e) = \left(V - X\left(X'V^{-1}X\right)^{-1}X'\right)\sigma^2 \tag{8.16}$$

8.5 Application of the WLS Model with Unequal Number of Subjects

Weighted least squares can be used when the number of subjects observed (r_i) is not the same for the i values of X. For example, for the averages ($\bar{y}_i$) calculated for the i values of X, the variance of each mean will be σ^2/r_i. The matrix W producing constant variances, $\mathrm{Var}(e^*) = I\sigma^2$, will be

$$W = \begin{pmatrix} \sqrt{r_1} & 0 & \cdots & 0 \\ 0 & \sqrt{r_2} & \cdots & 0 \\ \vdots & \vdots & \ddots & \vdots \\ 0 & 0 & \cdots & \sqrt{r_n} \end{pmatrix}$$

In this example, the transformed variable is $y_i^* = \bar{y}_i/a_i = \bar{y}_i\sqrt{r_i}$, where $\bar{y}_i$ is the average for a value of X and r_i is the number of observations for this average (see Table 8.1). There are two alternatives for the estimation of $\hat{Y}$ for the different

Table 8.1 Example of the transformed variable X using the number of subjects observed (r_i) for the weighting factor.

x_i	$\bar{y}_i$	r_i	$w_i = 1/a_i = \sqrt{r_i}$	$x_i^* = x_i/a_i = x_i\sqrt{r_i}$	$\bar{y}_i^* = \bar{y}_i/a_i = \bar{y}_i\sqrt{r_i}$
1	3.6	9	3	$1 \times 3 = 3$	$3.6 \times 3 = 10.8$
2	13.5	4	2	$2 \times 2 = 4$	$13.5 \times 2 = 27$
3	20	1	1	$3 \times 1 = 3$	$20 \times 1 = 20$

values of X through the WLS method: (i) design without the intercept, and (ii) model with intercept and weighting factor.

8.5.1 Design without Intercept

Consider the study variables defined as follows:

$$ya = Y^* = Y\sqrt{r}$$
$$xa = X^* = X\sqrt{r}$$
$$w = \sqrt{r}$$

For variables so defined, it is possible to obtain estimates of the coefficients by the OLS using a transformation. To carry out this operation in STATA, it is necessary to define this model without intercept and with predictor variables: xa and w. The syntax in STATA is as follows: **reg ya xa w, noconst**. When this command is used with the data of the Table 8.1, the resulting WLS model is described in Table 8.2.

Table 8.2 WLS model with predictor variables: xa and w.

```
  Source |       SS           df       MS            Number of obs   =        3
---------+----------------------------            F( 2,  1)        =   113.24
   Model | 1240.16419          2   620.082097      Prob > F         =   0.0663
Residual |  5.47579029         1     5.47579029    R-squared        =   0.9956
---------+----------------------------            Adj R-squared    =   0.9868
   Total | 1245.63998          3   415.213328      Root MSE         =      2.34
```

ya	Coefficient	Std. Error	t	$P > |t|$	95% Coefficient Interval	
xa	8.92	1.00	8.88	0.07	−3.85	21.68
w	−5.14	1.57	−3.28	0.19	−25.02	14.75

Based on these estimates, the model would be

$$\hat{y}_i^* = -5.14X_{0i}^* + 8.92X_{1i}^*$$

Therefore, the expected values on the model are

x	y	xa	ya	yaesp	yesp1
1.00	3.60	3.00	10.80	11.34	3.78
2.00	13.50	4.00	27.00	25.39	12.69
3.00	20.00	3.00	20.00	21.61	21.61

where

> *yaesp* = expected value of the response variable transformed
> *yesp1* = expected value of the response variable on the original scale
> $yesp1 = w^{-1}(yaesp)$

8.5.2 Model with Intercept and Weighting Factor

Another alternative is to carry out the estimate defining the variable *r* as a weighting factor. The syntax in STATA is `reg y x [weight=r]`. The result of this command is displayed in Table 8.3.

The point estimate of the intercept in Table 8.3 is exactly the same estimate of the coefficient of **w** in Table 8.2. In addition, the estimate of the coefficient of **x** in Table 8.3 is exactly the same estimate of the coefficient of **xa** in Table 8.2.

Table 8.3 WLS model with predictor variables *x* and using *r* as a weighting factor.

```
  Source |       SS       df       MS              Number of obs =        3
---------+------------------------------           F( 1,  1)      =    78.81
   Model | 92.4694751     1   92.4694751           Prob > F       =   0.0714
Residual | 1.17338352     1   1.17338352           R-squared      =   0.9875
---------+------------------------------           Adj R-squared  =   0.9749
   Total | 93.6428586     2   46.8214293           Root MSE       =   1.0832
```

y	Coefficient	Std. error	t	P > |t|	95% Coefficient interval	
x	8.92	1.00	8.88	0.07	−3.85	21.68
_cons	−5.14	1.57	−3.28	0.19	−25.02	14.75

8.6 Applications of the WLS Model When Variance Increases

This method can also be applied when the variance of Y increases as X increases, under the assumption that the regression model is conditional upon the values of X. In this situation, the matrix W producing constant variances, $\text{Var}(e^*) = I\sigma^2$, is

$$
W = \begin{pmatrix}
1/\sqrt{x_1} & 0 & \cdots & 0 \\
0 & 1/\sqrt{x_2} & \cdots & 0 \\
\vdots & \vdots & \ddots & \vdots \\
0 & 0 & \cdots & 1/\sqrt{x_n}
\end{pmatrix}
$$

The transformation of the variable Y will be $y_i^* = y_i/a_i = y_i/\sqrt{X_i}$. For example, given the following data,

X	Y
12	78
23	95
45	124
61	130
56	120
78	150
85	160

Two alternatives may be used to estimate $\hat{Y}$.

8.6.1 First Alternative

To carry out the estimation by the *OLS method*, under the assumption that Y increases as X increases, the transformation of the variables is as follows:

$$
ya = Y^* = Y/\sqrt{X}, \quad xa = X^* = X/\sqrt{X}, \quad \text{and} \quad w = 1/\sqrt{X}
$$

The estimation of the parameters when you run the simple regression model without the intercept (**reg ya xa w, noconst**) is described in Table 8.4. Based on these estimates, the model would be

$$
\hat{y}_i^* = 66.9X_{0i}^* + 1.08X_{1i}^*
$$

Table 8.4 WLS model when variance increases with predictor variables: *xa* and *w*.

```
Source |      SS        df      MS              Number of obs  =        7
-------+----------------------------            F(2, 5)        = 1690.74
 Model | 2361.41855     2   1180.70928          Prob > F       =  0.0000
Residual| 3.49170226    5   .698340453          R-squared      =  0.9985
-------+----------------------------            Adj R-squared  =  0.9979
 Total | 2364.91026     7   337.844322          Root MSE       =  .83567
```

ya	Coefficient	Std. error	t	P > |t|	95% Coefficient interval	
xa	1.08	0.07	14.40	0.00	0.89	1.27
w	66.91	3.12	21.45	0.00	58.89	74.93

The estimates of the expected values under this model are as follows:

x	y	xa	ya	yaesp	yesp1
12	78	3.464102	22.51666	23.05538	79.8662
23	95	4.795832	19.80887	19.12921	91.74048
45	124	6.708204	18.48483	17.21609	115.489
61	130	7.81025	16.64479	16.99827	132.7607
56	120	7.483315	16.03568	17.01964	127.3633
78	150	8.83176	16.98416	17.11005	151.1119
85	160	9.219544	17.35444	17.20999	158.6683

where

$yaesp$ = expected value of the response variable transformed
$yesp1$ = expected value of the response variable on the original scale
$$yesp1 = w^{-1}(yaesp)$$

8.6.2 Second Alternative

The second alternative is to perform the estimation defining the inverse of $X(1/X)$ as a weighting factor. The results are described in Table 8.5 and are similar to those presented in Tables 8.4.

Table 8.5 WLS model when variance increases and using $(1/X)$ as a weighting factor.

```
  Source |       SS        df       MS           Number of obs   =        7
---------+------------------------------         F(1, 5)         =   207.37
   Model |   4876.65006     1   4876.65006       Prob > F        =   0.0000
Residual |   117.582969     5   23.5165937       R-squared       =   0.9765
---------+------------------------------         Adj R-squared   =   0.9717
   Total |   4994.23303     6   832.372172       Root MSE        =   4.8494
```

ya	Coefficient	Std. error	t	P > |t|	95% Coefficient interval	
xa	1.08	0.07	14.40	0.000	0.89	1.27
w	66.91	3.12	21.45	0.000	58.89	74.93

Therefore, expected values are equal to the previous alternative:

x	y	yesp1	yesp2
12	78	79.9	79.9
23	95	91.7	91.7
45	124	115.5	115.5
61	130	132.8	132.8
56	120	127.4	127.4
78	150	151.1	151.1
85	160	158.7	158.7

where

$yesp1$ = expected value of the response variable using the first alternative

$yesp2$ = expected value of the response variable using the second alternative

8.7 Conclusions

This chapter presents two methods to achieve homogeneity of variance: the basic assumption for estimating the parameters of a multiple linear regression model using the OLS method. Situations that can cause deviation from variance homogeneity include (i) different number of observations for each value of X, and (ii) increase in the variance of Y as X increases (or decreases). Nonnormality and dependent observations may also lead to a violation of the constant variance. When a violation of normality and constant variance assumptions are suspected, a transformation of Y can help meet these assumptions. Weighted least-squares estimates of the coefficients will usually be nearly the same as the OLS estimates. In cases where they differ substantially, the procedure can be iterated until estimated coefficients stabilize. Often no more than one or two iterations are needed. In some cases, the values of the weights may be based on theory or prior research. In designed experiments with large numbers of replicates, weights can be estimated directly from sample variances of the response variable for each combination of the predictor variables. For more information on weighted least-squares estimation, please refer to Shin (2013).

Practice Exercise

Suppose we are interested in predicting the weight in premature children by gestational age. The following table presents the average weight (in grams) and the gestational age (in weeks) of 100 children with low birth weight.

Weight	Gestation	r
670.0	23	2
795.0	24	2
715.7	25	7
907.0	26	5
981.4	27	14
1075.5	28	11
1141.5	29	20
1151.5	30	13
1257.3	31	11
1266.0	32	5
1368.8	33	8
1440.0	34	1
1490.0	35	1

r indicates the number of births that had the same period of gestation.

a) Fit a regression model to explain the weight by gestational age without using the number of births as a weighting factor.

b) Using the previous model, display the residuals against the fitted values.

c) Fit a regression model to explain the weight as a function of gestational age using the number of births as a weighting factor.

d) Using the previous model, display the residuals against the fitted values.

References

Shin, H.C. (2013) Weighted least squares estimation with sampling weights. *Proceedings of the Survey Research Methods Section.* Alexandria, VA: The American Statistical Association.

9

Generalized Linear Models

Aim: Upon completing this chapter, the reader should be able to describe generalized linear models and their applications in epidemiology.

9.1 Introduction

The previous chapters have covered regression methods when the response variable is continuous. It is not hard to envision situations when the response variable is a discrete random variable, or even categorical. For example, number of obesity-related comorbidities, HIV status (positive or negative), blood pressure classification (normal, prehypertension, stage I hypertension, and stage II hypertension), and classification of weight status (underweight, normal, overweight, and obesity). Statistical regression can be conceptualized to include these types of response random variables through generalized linear models (GLM). These models attempt to fit a linear combination of predictors to a function of the expected value of a random variable. According to the characteristics of the random variables, we focus on the following representations of a GLM: (i) a classical regression model, (ii) a logistic regression model, and (iii) a Poisson regression model. This chapter describes GLM and their applications in epidemiology.

9.2 Specific Objectives

- Describe the application of GLM in different epidemiological designs.
- Identify the components of a GLM:
  - Random component
  - Systematic component
  - Link function
- Describe the general process of statistical hypothesis testing using GLM.

Applications of Regression Models in Epidemiology, First Edition. Erick Suárez, Cynthia M. Pérez, Roberto Rivera, and Melissa N. Martínez.
© 2017 John Wiley & Sons, Inc. Published 2017 by John Wiley & Sons, Inc.

9.3 Exponential Family of Probability Distributions

For a random variable Y, whose probability distribution is a function of a parameter of interest, there are various probability distributions that can be represented as follows (Nelder and Wedderburn, 1972; McCullagh and Nelder, 1989):

$$f(y; \theta) = e^{y \cdot \theta - b(\theta) + c(y)} \tag{9.1}$$

where

> θ is a function of the natural parameter of the probability distribution of Y. In case of the binomial distribution, $\theta = \ln(p/(1-p))$; for the Poisson distribution $\theta = \text{Ln}(\lambda)$; and for the normal distribution $\theta = \mu$.
>
> $b(\cdot), c(\cdot)$ are functions that vary according to the type of probability distribution associated with the random variable Y.
>
> e is the Euler constant, whose value is approximately 2.7183.

This representation identifies an exponential family of distributions, also known as EF (*exponential family*). Parameters other than the one of interest are considered nuisance parameters and can be placed in $b(\cdot)$, or $c(\cdot)$, and treated as known.

9.3.1 Binomial Distribution

The binomial distribution with parameter p belongs to the exponential family of distributions since it can be expressed as follows:

$$f(y; p) = \frac{n!}{y!(n-y)!} p^y (1-p)^{n-y}$$

$$f(y; p) = \exp\left[y \cdot \ln\left(\frac{p}{1-p}\right) + n \cdot \ln(1-p) + \ln\left(\frac{n!}{y!(n-y)!}\right) \right] \tag{9.2}$$

where

$\theta = \ln\left(\frac{p}{1-p}\right)$

$b(\theta) = -n \cdot \ln(1-p) = n \cdot \ln(1 + \exp(\theta))$

$c(y) = \ln\left(\frac{n!}{y!(n-y)!}\right)$

Y is the number of "successes" in n Bernoulli experiments

$\quad p = $ Probability of success at every trial.

An example of a binomial random variable is the number of pregnant women with complications during labor out of 100 pregnant women randomly chosen.

9.3.2 Poisson Distribution

The Poisson distribution with distribution parameter λ also belongs to the exponential family of distributions because it can be expressed as follows:

$$f(y; \lambda) = \frac{\lambda^y e^{-\lambda}}{y!} = \exp\left(y \ln(\lambda) - \lambda - \ln(y!)\right) \tag{9.3}$$

where

$$\theta = \ln(\lambda)$$
$$b(\theta) = \lambda = \exp(\theta)$$
$$c(y) = -\ln(y!)$$
$$\lambda = E(Y)$$

λ is the average number of persons with a specific characteristic during a certain period. An example is the average number of new cases of lung cancer reported every year.

9.4 Exponential Family of Probability Distributions with Dispersion

The exponential family of probability distributions can be generalized by including a constant or a scaling parameter ϕ as follows:

$$f(y; \theta, \phi) = e^{[y \cdot \theta - b(\theta)/(a(\phi))] + c(y, \phi)} \tag{9.4}$$

This type of distribution is classified as a family of exponential distributions with dispersion (*exponential dispersion family*), also known as EDF. Usually, $a(\phi)$ is represented by ϕ/w, where w is a weighting factor for each observation. If the function $a(\phi)$ is equal to unity, $a(\phi) = 1$, then the resultant EDF is an EF of probability distributions. If ϕ is known, we define a special case of EDF with a single parameter (Lindsey, 1997). One of the distributions of continuous random variables with an EDF representation is the normal distribution, since its *density function* satisfies the following condition:

$$f(y; \mu, \sigma^2) = \frac{1}{\sqrt{2\pi\sigma^2}} e^{-((y-\mu)^2/2\sigma^2)}$$
$$= e^{\left[\frac{y \cdot \mu - (\mu^2/2)}{\sigma^2} - \frac{y^2}{2\sigma^2} - \frac{1}{2}\ln(2\pi\sigma^2)\right]} \tag{9.5}$$

where

$$\theta = \mu$$
$$b(\theta) = \theta^2/2$$
$$a(\phi) = \sigma^2$$
$$c(y, \phi) = -\frac{1}{2}\left[\frac{y^2}{a(\phi)} + \ln(2\pi a(\phi))\right]$$

μ is the mean value of Y and σ is the standard deviation of Y. For an example, μ could be the mean value of cholesterol levels and σ the standard deviation of cholesterol levels.

In case where Y is defined as the average of m independent measurements with normal distribution, the function $a(\phi)$ would be

$$a(\phi) = \frac{\sigma^2}{m}$$

where the weights, in this case, correspond to the total number of measurements used to obtain the average ($w = m$).

9.5 Mean and Variance in EF and EDF

For members of EF and EDF, there is a special relationship between the mean and the variance of the random variable Y (Lindsey, 1997):

i) Mean of Y (expected value of Y)

$$E(Y) = b'(\theta) = \frac{\partial b(\theta)}{\partial \theta} = \begin{cases} np, & \text{in the case of a binomial distribution} \\ \lambda, & \text{in the case of a Poisson distribution} \\ \mu, & \text{in the case of a normal distribution} \end{cases}$$

The term $\partial b(\theta)/\partial \theta$ indicates the first partial derivative of the function $b(\theta)$ with respect to θ (Swokowski, 2000). This relationship applies to the probability distributions of the EF and also to the probability distributions of the EDF.

ii) Variance of Y

$$\mathrm{Var}(Y) = E\left[(Y - E(Y))^2\right] = a(\phi) \cdot \frac{\partial^2 b(\theta)}{\partial \theta^2} = a(\phi) \cdot \tau^2$$

where $\partial^2 b(\theta)/\partial \theta^2 = b''(\theta)$ indicates the second derivative of the function $b(\theta)$ with respect to θ. As a consequence, the variance of Y in EDF distributions will depend of the product of the dispersion parameter, ϕ, and the parameter τ^2. The symbol τ^2 is defined as the variance function, which results in different expressions depending on the distribution of the random variable Y (see Table 9.1).

Table 9.1 Variance function by distribution type.

Distribution	Variance function, τ^2
Binomial	$np(1 - p)$
Poisson	λ
Normal	1

9.6 Definition of a Generalized Linear Model

A GLM establishes a relationship between a function of the expected value of a random variable and a set of variables expressed as a linear combination of the following form:

$$\eta_i = g(E(Y_i)) = \beta_0 + \beta_1 X_1 + \cdots + \beta_m X_m \tag{9.6}$$

where Y_i is a variable with probability distribution from the EF or EDF and the index i indicates a specific combination of the values of the predictor variables X_i. The basic components of a GLM are as follows:

- **Random Component**. This is a random variable Y with mean or expected value $E(Y_i)$.
- **Link Function**. This is a function of the expected value of the random variable, $E(Y_i)$, usually identified by the Greek letter $\eta_i = g(E(Y_i))$.
- **Systematic Component**. This is a linear combination of the predictor variables expressed, as follows:

$$\beta_0 + \beta_1 X_1 + \cdots + \beta_m X_m$$

The objective of a GLM is to determine the relationship between η and a set of predictors. The effect of each predictor on η depends on the estimated value of the corresponding β coefficient. Moreover, the link function that is used in a GLM depends on the probability distribution of the dependent variable (see Table 9.2).

When the link function is the identity function, the GLM identifies a linear regression model. If the link function is the natural logarithm, the GLM identifies a Poisson regression model. If the link function is the logit, the GLM identifies a logistic regression model. The *canonical link function* uses the parameter of the probability distribution of the random variable. For example, for the Poisson distribution, the canonical link is the natural logarithm of the mean, while for the binomial distribution it is the logit function of the probability of success:

$$\ln \left(\frac{p_i}{1 - p_i} \right)$$

Table 9.2 Link function by distribution type.

Probability distribution in Y	Link function	
Binomial	$\eta_i = \ln \left(\frac{E(Y_i)}{1 - E(Y_i)} \right)$	Logit (Logit function)
Poisson	$\eta_i = \ln(E(Y_i))$	Natural logarithm
Normal	$\eta_i = E(Y_i)$	Identity

9.7 Estimation Methods

The estimation of the β coefficients in the GLM is done using the *maximum likelihood* method. Suppose we have a random sample $y_1, \ldots, y_n$ from m subjects or units of study (e.g., families, hospitals, and clinics). The joint density function for all observations can be written as $f(y_1, \ldots, y_n | \psi)$, where ψ is a vector of distribution parameters. The likelihood function is essentially the joint distribution as a function ψ for fixed observations. The maximum likelihood method determines the parameter values that maximize the likelihood function that relates ψ to the observed values of the random variables $Y_1, \ldots, Y_n$. The likelihood function is represented as follows:

$$L = f(Y_1, \ldots, Y_n | \psi) \tag{9.7}$$

Under the assumption that the observations are independent, the likelihood function is defined by the following expression:

$$L = f(Y_1 | \psi) f(Y_2 | \psi) \cdots f(Y_n | \psi)$$

The specific definition of $f(Y_i | \psi)$ for $i = 1, \ldots, n$ depends on the probability distribution of the random variable Y_i. In the case of the binomial distribution, the likelihood function is defined as follows:

$$L = f(Y_1 | n_i, p_i)^* \ldots {}^* f(Y_1 | n_i, p_i) = \prod_{i=1}^{n} \frac{n_i}{y_i! (n_i - y_i)!} p_i^{y_i} (1 - p_i)^{(n_i - y_i)} \tag{9.8}$$

where the parameter p_i is the success probability of the binomial distribution or the binomial proportion, and n_i is the number of subjects in ith group. With the GLM, the p_i can be expressed in terms of a set of m predictors as follows:

$$p_i = \frac{1}{1 + e^{-\left(\beta_0 + \sum_{j=1}^{m} \beta_j X_{i,j}\right)}} \tag{9.9}$$

or

$$\text{logit}(p_i) = \ln\left(\frac{p_i}{1 - p_i}\right) = \beta_0 + \sum_{j=1}^{m} \beta_j X_{i,j}$$

Therefore, the likelihood function is reconfigured, that is, the new parameters of L are the coefficients β_i associated with the predictor variables, X_i, as follows:

$$L = \prod_{i=1}^{n} \frac{n_i}{y_i! (n_i - y_i)!} \left(\frac{1}{1 + e^{-\left(\beta_0 + \sum_{j=1}^{m} \beta_j X_{i,j}\right)}}\right)^{y_i} \left(1 - \frac{1}{1 + e^{-\left(\beta_0 + \sum_{j=1}^{m} \beta_j X_{i,j}\right)}}\right)^{(n_i - y_i)} \tag{9.10}$$

To facilitate the estimation of $\beta_i (i = 1, \ldots, n)$, it is usually more desirable to maximize the natural logarithm of L, $\ln(L)$, since the estimators of β_i that maximize $\ln(L)$ also maximize L (Collett, 2002). The estimates of β_i are obtained via the maximum likelihood method using the following equations (*score equations*):

$$\frac{\partial \ln(L)}{\partial \beta_j} = 0 \text{ for } j = 0, 1, \ldots, m$$

subject to the condition:

$$\frac{\partial^2 \ln(L)}{\partial \beta_j^2} < 0$$

The result of these equations depends on the type of probability distribution used. These equations are usually solved using iterative methods, which use an initial value in the possible solution β^0, to generate another solution β^1. This process continues until the difference between two consecutive solutions does not exceed a preset value. When using the maximum likelihood method, caution is needed because it can produce biased estimates. In case of large samples, the maximum likelihood estimates are the estimates with the minimum variance and are normally distributed, regardless of the original distribution of the data (Collett, 2002).

9.8 *Deviance* Calculation

To evaluate the significance of the estimates of the regression coefficients (β_i), obtained by the maximum likelihood method, a comparison is performed between the following two likelihood functions:

i) Likelihood based on the estimated parameters from the model of interest (L_c)
ii) Likelihood with a parameter for every observation (L_f). This is also known as the saturated model and provides a perfect fit to the data.

The distance between the observed y_i and the fitted $\hat{y}_i$ defines the *residual deviance* or *deviance*, which is computed using the natural logarithm of the ratio of these likelihood functions (*log-likelihood ratio*), as follows:

$$D = -2 \ln \left(\frac{L_c}{L_f}\right) = -2[\ln(L_c) - \ln(L_f)] \tag{9.11}$$

The formula of this measure varies according to the probability distribution associated with the dependent variable under study. Table 9.3 presents the

Table 9.3 Deviance by probability distribution.

Probability distribution	Deviance
Binomial	$2\sum_{i=1}^{n}\left[y_i \ln\left(\dfrac{y_i}{n_i\hat{p}_i}\right) + (n_i - y_i)\ln\left(\dfrac{n_i - y_i}{n_i - n\hat{p}_i}\right)\right]$
Poisson	$2\sum_{i=1}^{n}\left[y_i \ln\left(\dfrac{y_i}{\hat{\lambda}_i}\right) - (y_i - \hat{\lambda}_i)\right]$
Normal	$\sum_{i=1}^{n}(y_i - \hat{\mu}_i)^2$

different formulas for *deviance* by type of probability distribution associated with the dependent variable.

where

y_i indicates the observed value of the dependent variable.
n_i indicates the number of observations in the group i.
ln indicates the natural logarithm function.
$\hat{\mu}_i$ indicates the estimate of the expected value of y_i under the model.
$\hat{\lambda}_i$ indicates the rate estimate i under the model.
$\hat{p}_i$ indicates the estimate of the proportion i under the model.

To determine the adequacy of the model for explaining Y when it has a binomial or Poisson distribution, the relationship between the *deviance* and degrees of freedom should be assessed. Under a suitable model,

$$\text{Deviance} \approx \text{Degrees of freedom}$$

This relationship can be formally tested since the *deviance* will follow a chi-square distribution, χ^2_{df}. In addition, the deviance will enable both statistical testing and model comparisons.

9.9 Hypothesis Evaluation

To determine the effect of the predictor variables, it is necessary to evaluate the changes in the *deviance* when comparing the model with all the predictors against a reduced model of a subset of predictors (a nested model such as a model without predictors). The null hypothesis will be defined by the coefficients of the predictors that were removed from the full model.

For example, assume the following two models:

$$\text{Full model}: \eta_i = \beta_0 + \beta_1 X_1 + \beta_2 X_2 + \beta_3 X_3$$

$$\text{Incomplete or reduced model}: \eta'_i = \beta_0 + \beta_1 X_1$$

Comparing the corresponding *deviances* will evaluate the hypothesis $H_0 : \beta_2 = \beta_3 = 0_{|X_1}$; that is, the coefficients of X_2 and X_3 are assumed to be zero when X_1 is present in the model. In an epidemiological study the variable X_1 may represent the exposure variable, whereas X_2 and X_3 may represent potential confounding variables.

The specific method for comparing the respective *deviances* will depend on the probability distribution associated with the random variable under consideration. Table 9.4 identifies the statistic to evaluate the null hypothesis, H_0, depending on the type of probability distribution.

D_{CM} : indicates the *deviance* with all independent variables (full model).
D_{INC} : indicates the *deviance* with a subset of independent variables (incomplete model).
df_{CM} : indicates the degrees of freedom reported for the full model *deviance.*
df_{INC} : indicates the degrees of freedom reported for the incomplete model *deviance.*

The comparison of the two deviances $(LR = D_{INC} - D_{CM})$ is called the *likelihood ratio test statistic*. For large samples, the LR test statistic follows approximately a χ^2 distribution with degrees of freedom equal to the difference between the degrees of freedom of each model.

To evaluate an individual predictor, $H_0 : \beta_i = 0_{|X_1,X_2,...,X_{i-1},X_{i+1},...,X_k}$, an alternative to the LR test statistic is the *Wald* test, which involves the estimated parameter β_i and its corresponding standard error, as follows:

$$W = \left(\frac{\hat{\beta}_i}{se(\hat{\beta}_i)} \right)^2 \sim \chi^2_{(1)} \tag{9.12}$$

where $se(\hat{\beta}_i)$ is the asymptotic (i.e., large sample) standard error of the $\hat{\beta}_i$. For large enough n, W is distributed as χ^2 with 1 df. The statistic $\sqrt{W}$

Table 9.4 Test statistic in the assessment of H_0.

Probability distribution	Test statistic	Probability distribution to assess the test statistic
Binomial	$\chi^2_c = D_{INC} - D_{CM}$	Chi-square $\chi^2(df_{INC} - df_{CM})$
Poisson	$\chi^2_c = D_{INC} - D_{CM}$	Chi-square $\chi^2(df_{INC} - df_{CM})$
Normal	$F_c = \dfrac{(D_{INC} - D_{CM})/(df_{INC} - df_{CM})}{D_{MC}/df_{CM}}$	F-Fisher $F_{(df_{INC}-df_{CM},df_{CM})}$

asymptotically follows a standard normal distribution under the null hypothesis. Several statistical software treat $\sqrt{W}$ as having a t-distribution instead of a normal distribution. In OLR models, the t-distribution is used to account for the fact that the variance of $Y|X$ is estimated. However, in a model with a binomial outcome, there is not a separate variance parameter to estimate. An asymptotic $100(1 - \alpha)\%$ confidence intervals for β_i is given by

$$\hat{\beta}_i \pm Z_{(1-\alpha/2)}\text{se}\left(\hat{\beta}_i\right) \tag{9.13}$$

Wald-based confidence intervals are also symmetric even though the coverage probability may not be (Harrell, 2015; Fox, 2008).

9.10 Analysis of Residuals

There are different types of residuals encountered in GLM and they are generally similar to the various types of residuals defined for the OLR model in Chapter 7. The response or raw residuals are simply given by

$$\hat{e}_i = y_i - \hat{y}_i \tag{9.14}$$

The Pearson residuals are defined as

$$\hat{e}_{P,i} = \sqrt{\phi}\,\frac{y_i - \hat{y}_i}{\sqrt{\hat{V}(y_i)}} \tag{9.15}$$

If $\phi \neq 1$, the residuals may be multiplied by $\sqrt{\phi}$ or its estimates to produce scaled versions of these residuals. Based on these residuals, the Pearson χ^2 statistic is defined as

$$\chi^2 = \chi^2\left(y_i, \hat{y}_i\right) = \sum_{i=1}^{n} \hat{e}_{P,i}^2$$

which is asymptotically equivalent to the deviance D.

The deviance residuals are defined as

$$\hat{e}_{D,i} = sign\left(y_i - \hat{y}_i\right)^* 2w_i^* \left[y_i\left(\theta(y_i) - \hat{\theta}_i\right) - \left(b\left(\theta(y_i)\right) - b\left(\hat{\theta}_i\right)\right)\right] \tag{9.16}$$

where w_i is a weighting factor for each observation. This definition ensures that $\sum_{i=1}^{n} \hat{e}_{D,i}^2 = D$.

Plots of residuals can be used to check model adequacy by plotting residuals against individual covariates or against the $\hat{y}_i$ or the $\hat{\eta}_i$. However, caution should be taken for Poisson data because small counts may cause naturally occurring patterns in the residuals, which should not be interpreted as indicating model inadequacy (Bingham and Fry, 2010).

9.11 Model Selection

There are several criteria to select the predictors of a GLM, such as the AIC and BIC introduced in sections 5.4.5 and 5.4.6. In epidemiological study designs, elimination of predictors does not necessarily depend on statistical significance criteria. The main statistical goal in these designs is to determine the magnitude of the association between the exposure factor and a disease controlling the effect of potential confounding variables (Kleinbaum et al., 2014).

The definition of the final model will depend on the design of the study being used. In a descriptive epidemiological study the final model is defined usually by a fixed number of predictors of interest, based on the scientific literature, or by a small group of these variables using some elimination criteria (i.e., backward, forward, and stepwise). In an analytical epidemiological study, the final model is defined by the exposure variable plus a set of confounding and interaction variables; the exposure variable is never eliminated. When no interaction variables are included in the model, potential confounding variables should remain in the GLM to estimate the adjusted magnitude of the association between the exposure factor and a study disease. In the following chapters, this procedure will be applied for the classical epidemiological designs.

9.12 Bayesian Models

Bayesian methodology is applied in a GLM by assuming a prior distribution for each of the β coefficients:

$$\eta_i = \beta_0 + \beta_1 X_1 + \beta_2 X_2 + \beta_3 X_3$$

where $\beta_i \sim \psi(\kappa_i)$ and $\psi(\kappa_i)$ indicate the prior distribution with its parameters κ_i.

The goal is to obtain *credible intervals* for posterior probabilities of the predictions or the model coefficients. These intervals are usually obtained through Monte Carlo simulations (Congdon, 2005).

One of the difficulties of Bayesian methods is the selection of the prior distribution, and one commonly used alternative is the uniform distribution. Another difficulty is how to obtain a specific formula for the posterior distribution, and hence simulation techniques have been used frequently. This process requires the use of specialized statistical software, such as Win-BUGS, though newer versions of different statistical software, such as Stata and SAS, have incorporated this type of analysis. For more information on the application of these methods, refer to Woodward (2014).

9.13 Conclusions

Generalized linear models have been an important development for epidemiology. They have been the main instruments of statistical analysis in the evaluation of the association between an outcome of interest and an exposure, controlling for potential confounding variables. In addition, these models are used to estimate the magnitude of the association between an exposure and a disease, adjusted for confounders, as we will see in the following chapters.

How to quantify the association of disease and exposure varies according to the epidemiological study design. In a case-control study, the measure of association is the *odds ratio*, which can be estimated by the logistic regression model. In a cohort study, the classical measure of association is the relative risk, which can be estimated by the Poisson regression model. For cross-sectional designs, the measure of association is the prevalence ratio, which can be estimated using the logistic regression model or with the Poisson regression model (Gordis, 2014).

References

Bingham, N.H. and Fry, J.M. (2010) *Regression Linear Models in Statistics*, London, UK: Springer.

Collett, D. (2002) *Modelling Binary Data*, 2nd edition. London: Chapman & Hall.

Congdon, P. (2005) *Bayesian Models for Categorical Data*, Chichester: John Wiley & Sons, Ltd.

Fox, J. (2008) *Applied Regression Analysis and Generalized Linear Models*, 2nd edition. Thousand Oaks, CA: Sage Publications.

Gordis, L. (2014) *Epidemiology*, 5th edition. Philadelphia, PA: Elsevier Saunders.

Harrell, F.E. (2015) *Regression Modeling Strategies with Applications to Linear Models, Logistic and Ordinal Regression, and Survival Analysis*, 2nd edition. New York, NY: Springer.

Kleinbaum, D.G., Kupper, L.L., Nizam, A., and Rosenberg, E.S. (2014) *Applied Regression Analysis and Other Multivariable Methods*, 5th edition. Boston, MA: Cengage Learning.

Lindsey, J.K. (1997) *Applying Generalized Linear Models*. New York, NY: Springer.

McCullagh, P. and Nelder, J. (1989) *Generalized Linear Models*, 2nd edition. Boca Raton, FL: Chapman & Hall.

Nelder, J.A. and Wedderburn, R.W.M. (1972) Generalized linear models. *J. R. Statist. Soc. A*, **135**, 370–384.

Swokowski, E. (2000) *Calculus: The Classic Edition*, 5th edition. Cengage Advantage Books.

Woodward, M. (2014) *Epidemiology: Study Design and Data Analysis*, 3rd edition. Boca Raton, FL: Chapman & Hall.

10

Poisson Regression Models for Cohort Studies

Aim: Upon completing this chapter, the reader should be able to fit a generalized linear model for a count response in a cohort study design.

10.1 Introduction

In a cohort study, a disease-free study population is selected on the basis of their exposure to a factor and followed over a period of time to determine the occurrence of disease or any other health-related event. The incidence of disease is then compared in exposed and unexposed groups (see Figure 10.1).

Cohort studies are classified as prospective (concurrent) or historical (retrospective), depending on the time when information about the exposure is collected. In a prospective cohort study, subjects are classified based on their exposure status at the beginning of the study; in a historical cohort study, determination of the exposure status is made for the past, and assessed using preexisting records that are accurate and complete. In either design, the statistical goal is to estimate disease incidence among exposed and unexposed individuals prior to quantifying the magnitude of the association between exposure and disease.

The main methodological advantage of a cohort design is that the temporal sequence between the exposure under study and the disease or any other health-related event can be established (Gordis, 2014). Other important advantages of this design include determination of disease incidence in each exposure group and investigation of the effect of the exposure of interest on multiple outcomes. One major disadvantage of this design is its susceptibility to loss of subjects during follow-up, which may introduce selection bias and thus affect the internal validity of the study (Gordis, 2014). Thus, comparability of subjects who remain in the study until disease occurrence or the study is completed and those who are lost to follow-up, by exposure status, must be determined in order to assess potential selection bias.

Applications of Regression Models in Epidemiology, First Edition. Erick Suárez,
Cynthia M. Pérez, Roberto Rivera, and Melissa N. Martínez.
© 2017 John Wiley & Sons, Inc. Published 2017 by John Wiley & Sons, Inc.

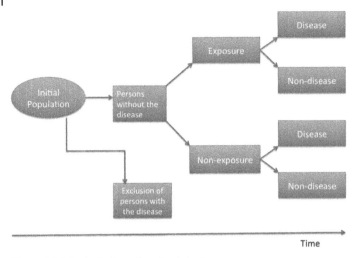

Figure 10.1 Basic design of a cohort study.

10.2 Specific Objectives

- Describe the different measures of incidence in a cohort study.
- Define the concept of crude and adjusted relative risk (RR) using a Poisson regression model.
- Assess confounding and interaction effects using a Poisson regression model.

10.3 Incidence Measures

Incidence is an epidemiological measure that quantifies the number of new cases of a disease that develop in a population at risk during a specific time period. There are two main measures that are used to quantify incidence: incidence density and cumulative incidence (CI).

10.3.1 Incidence Density

The incidence rate is determined by the relationship between the occurrence of new cases and the population exposed at each instant of time (Selvin, 2004). Because it is almost impossible to express the study population as a function of time, only rarely can you get the incidence rate. Szklo and Nieto (2007) define incidence density as the number of events per person time, based on a cohort for which individual data and the exact follow-up time for each individual are available over a period of time (t_0, t). Incidence density (ID) is expressed

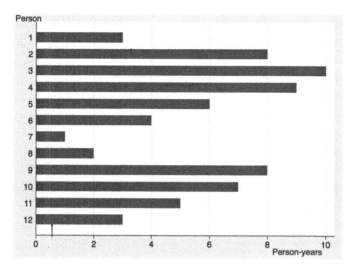

Figure 10.2 Determination of person-years in a hypothetical study.

mathematically as follows:

$$\text{ID} = \frac{a}{L} = \frac{\text{New cases in a period}}{\sum_{i=1}^{n} \Delta t_i} \qquad (10.1)$$

where Δt_i is the individual follow-up time, which is calculated based on the difference between the date when the participant joined the study and the date of occurrence of the disease or the date of loss to follow-up. Usually, the cumulative follow-up time over all individuals (usually expressed in person-years, person-semesters, or person-days) for the population observed during the study period (Figure 10.2). To facilitate interpretation of incidence density, this measure is usually multiplied by a constant (10^k). In practice, the average incidence density is often used interchangeably with incidence rate.

Figure 10.2 illustrates the computation of person-years using a hypothetical cohort of 12 subjects observed for a period of 10 years. Three developed the disease (4, 6, and 7). The total person-years (66 person-years) is the sum of the individual time at risk of all subjects. Based on this information, the average incidence density during the study period is given by

$$\text{ID} = \frac{3}{3 + 5 + \cdots + 3} = \frac{3}{66 \text{ person-years}} = 4.54 \text{ per } 100 \text{ person-years}$$

This result indicates that there were 3 cases of disease during 66 person-years of follow-up or 4.54 cases of disease during 100 person-years. The concept of "100 person-years" may be equivalent to 100 healthy individuals observed over a year. One can also express this result as on average 4.54 new cases of disease per

Table 10.1 Classical notation for estimating the incidence density.

	Exposure	Nonexposure
Number of new cases	a_1	a_0
Person-years	L_1	L_0
Incidence density	$ID_1 = a_1/L_1$	$ID_0 = a_0/L_0$

Here a_i denotes the number of new cases in the ith group and L_i denotes the total accumulated person-years in the ith group.

100 persons observed over a year. Table 10.1 presents the notation used to determine the incidence density in two groups (exposed and unexposed) in a cohort study.

Based on this notation, the relative risk is expressed as follows:

$$RR = \frac{ID_1}{ID_0} = \frac{a_1/L_1}{a_0/L_0} \tag{10.2}$$

When the RR takes the null value (RR = 1), it means that the incidence of disease in exposed and unexposed groups is the same. When the RR exceeds the null value (RR > 1), the incidence of disease is greater in the exposed group than in the unexposed group (exposure is associated with an increased risk of disease). If the RR is below the null value (RR < 1), then the incidence of disease is lower in the exposed group than in the unexposed group (exposure is associated with a reduction in risk of disease). To illustrate the calculation of the incidence density and the corresponding relative risk in a cohort study, we use the data described in Table 10.2.

Based on the data of Table 10.2, the incidence density of cardiovascular disease in the group of smokers is

$$\left(\frac{43}{727}\right) \times 1000 = 59.1 \times 1000$$

The incidence density of cardiovascular disease in the group of nonsmokers is

$$\left(\frac{52}{1820}\right) \times 1000 = 28.6 \times 1000$$

Table 10.2 Hypothetical data on the association between smoking and cardiovascular disease in a cohort study.

	Smokers	Nonsmokers
Number of newly diagnosed cases of cardiovascular disease	43	52
Person-years	727	1820

The results of this hypothetical study indicate the following:

i) For every 1000 smokers observed in a year, there were 59.1 cases of cardiovascular disease.

ii) For every 1000 nonsmokers observed in a year, there were 28.6 new cases of cardiovascular disease.

Therefore, the estimator of the relative risk is

$$\widehat{RR} = \frac{59.1}{28.6} = 2.06$$

This result indicates that smokers were 2.06 times as likely to develop cardiovascular disease as nonsmokers. Alternatively, smokers had 2.06 times the risk of cardiovascular disease compared to nonsmokers. Another approach to calculate the incidence density is to approximate the population at risk by the mid-year population, which is computed by averaging the populations at the beginning and end of the study period (Selvin, 2004) as follows:

$$ID = \frac{New\ cases}{\sum_{i=1}^{n} \Delta t_i} \approx \frac{New\ cases}{Mid\text{-year population}} \qquad (10.3)$$

10.3.2 Cumulative Incidence

When the period of observation of each subject in the cohort study is constant ($\Delta t_i = t$), the occurrence of a disease or health-related event is calculated using the cumulative incidence (also referred to as risk or incidence proportion). This measure is obtained with the following formula:

$$CI = \frac{New\ cases\ in\ a\ period}{n} \qquad (10.4)$$

where n indicates the population at risk at the start of the study. For example, assume that the objective of a cohort study is to evaluate the occurrence of complications during delivery among obese and nonobese pregnant women. To determine the cumulative incidence in this study, it is assumed that (a) there is no loss of follow-up in the study and (b) the observation period is approximately 9 months. In this case, the cumulative incidence in each group is

$$CI = \frac{Number\ of\ women\ who\ develop\ complications\ during\ delivery}{Women\ at\ risk\ at\ beginning\ of\ the\ study}$$

Table 10.3 shows the typical notation to estimate the cumulative incidence in a cohort study, when the exposure is dichotomous (exposed and unexposed).

Table 10.3 Typical notation to estimate cumulative incidence (CI).

	Exposed	Unexposed
New cases	a_1	a_0
Total	n_1	n_0
Cumulative incidence	$CI_1 = a_1/n_1$	$CI_0 = a_0/n_0$

Here a_i denotes the number of new cases at the end of the study in the ith group of exposure and n_i denotes the number of individuals at risk in the ith group of exposure.

Using the above notation, the relative risk (RR) is equivalent to the following expression:

$$RR = \frac{CI_1}{CI_0} = \frac{a_1/n_1}{a_0/n_0} \tag{10.5}$$

To illustrate the computation of the cumulative incidence, data from a hypothetical study on the impact of obesity in early pregnancy and the occurrence of complications during childbirth in 970 pregnant women are given in Table 10.4.

The results of this study indicate that, on average, 22.1% obese women experienced complications during childbirth, whereas 14.2% nonobese women had complications during childbirth. Therefore, obese women had 1.55 times the risk of childbirth complications than nonobese women. An alternative interpretation for this result is that obese women had 55% higher risk of having childbirth complications than nonobese women.

10.4 Confounding Variable

Confounding is a distortion in the estimated magnitude of association that is produced when an extraneous factor (unobserved exposure) is associated with the exposure of interest and with the disease or health-related event

Table 10.4 Hypothetical study on obesity and complications during childbirth.

Complications	Obese	Nonobese	Relative risk
Present	95	77	
Absent	335	463	
Total	430	540	$\hat{RR} = \frac{0.221}{0.142} = 1.55$
Cumulative incidence	$CI_1 = 0.221$	$CI_0 = 0.142$	

Figure 10.3 Example of a confounding variable.

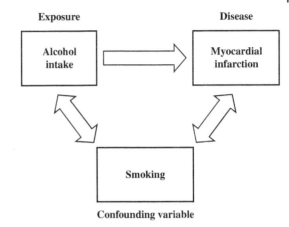

(see Figure 10.3). The confounding variable cannot be an intermediate step in the causal pathway between the exposure and disease or health-related event. Failure to control for the confounding variable, either in the design or analytical stages, might distort the magnitude of association as it can underestimate (negative confounding) or overestimate (positive confounding) the effect of the exposure on the outcome.

To evaluate the effect of potential confounding variables, it is necessary to compare the degree of discrepancy between the point estimate of the crude *relative risk* $(\hat{RR}_{crude})$ and the point estimate of the adjusted *relative risk* $(\hat{RR}_{adjusted})$. In general, if the $\hat{RR}_{crude}$ is similar to $\hat{RR}_{adjusted}$, it is concluded that the confounding variables have no effect on the magnitude of the association of interest. Otherwise, it is recommended to determine if the $\hat{RR}_{crude}$ overestimates or underestimates the association of interest using as a reference the $\hat{RR}_{adjusted}$.

10.5 Stratified Analysis

When we are interested in analyzing the magnitude of the association between exposure and disease while controlling for potential confounding variables, it is recommended to assess the association in different strata defined by levels of the confounding variables; for example, the association of smoking habit (exposure) and lung cancer (disease) at different age groups (strata). For each stratum, an RR is estimated for the association of interest. Then, these RRs are compared in order to assess effect modification. In the case where exposure is categorized in two groups, the *Mantel–Haenszel* method has been used to test the homogeneity of the RRs over different strata defined from levels of one or several confounding variables (Rothman et al., 2008). This method uses the following estimate of a common RR, which is valid when the RRs in each stratum are homogeneous:

$$\text{RR}_{\text{MH}} = \sum_{k=1}^{K} \frac{w_k \text{RR}_k}{w_k} \tag{10.6}$$

where K is the total number of strata, w_k is the weighted factor in the kth stratum, which is determined as the product of the number of cases who are unexposed and the total number of exposed divided by the number of subjects in this stratum. Further details on how to perform a test for homogeneity using different measures of association can be found in Jewell (2004). If the underlying (true) RR is different across the strata, then there is said to be interaction or effect modification between the exposure and a third variable or factor, which is called effect modifier (Rosner, 2010). Distinction between interaction and effect modification has already been made (VanderWeele, 2009). Interaction is defined in terms of the effects of two factors, whereas effect modification is defined in terms of the effect of one factor varying across strata of a second variable. However, the terms "interaction" and "effect modification" in practice are often used interchangeably.

10.6 Poisson Regression Model

The Poisson regression model estimates the incidence of a disease or health-related event under different conditions. To determine the incidence, it is necessary to compute the number of new cases during the observation period and identify the initial conditions of the study, such as the type of exposure at baseline and specific values of the potential confounding variables. The Poisson model establishes a relationship between the expected number of cases and the exposure while controlling for potential confounders, using the following exponential function:

$$\mu_i = P_i^* e^{\beta_0 + \beta_E E_i + \sum_{j=1}^{J} \beta_j C_j} \tag{10.7}$$

where

- μ_i indicates the expected value of new cases under the condition i. These conditions i indicate a combination of the values of the predictor variables (including exposure and of confounding variables). We assume that the number of new cases is a random variable that has a Poisson distribution.
- P_i indicates the population at baseline in the ith group of exposure. If P denotes person-time, then the model will estimate the incidence density; however, if P indicates the population at risk at baseline, the model will estimate the cumulative incidence.
- E_i indicates the exposure variable.

β_E indicates the regression coefficient associated with the exposure variable.

C_j indicates the jth confounding variable. We assume J indicates is the total number of potential confounding variables.

β_j indicates the regression coefficient associated with the jth confounding variable.

β_0 indicates the intercept of the model. The exponential of this value is the expected incidence of the number of new cases when the exposure and the confounding variables take the value of zero.

We are assuming that the response variable (Y) is in the form of a count occurring independently among different subgroups, such as the number of newly diagnosed cases of kidney cancer at different hospitals every 5 years. In addition, we assume that this random variable describes rare events and follows a Poisson distribution:

$$\Pr[Y = k] = \mu^k e^\mu / k! \tag{10.8}$$

where $E(Y) = \text{Var}(Y) = \mu$, and k is the specific value of Y (0,1,2, . . .).

In the Poisson model, we assume that μ is linked to the exponential of a linear function of the exposure variable and a set of confounding variables; so the changes in the incidence resulting from the combined effects of the exposure and the confounding variables are multiplicative:

$$\frac{\mu_i}{P_i} = e^{\beta_0 *} e^{\beta_E E *} e^{\sum_{j=1}^{J} \beta_j C_j} \tag{10.9}$$

An alternative to describing the Poisson regression model is given by the following expression:

$$\ln(\mu_i) = \ln(P_i) + \beta_0 + \beta_E E + \sum_{j=1}^{J} \beta_j C_j \tag{10.10}$$

The natural logarithm of the expected cases can be expressed as the natural logarithm of person-time or population at risk, as appropriate, plus a linear combination of the predictors. That is, the natural logarithm of the expected number of cases is represented by a generalized linear model, whose link function is the natural logarithm. Since the model contains the variable $\ln(P_i)$ with a coefficient equal to unity, there is no need to estimate the coefficient for this variable, referred to as an *offset* variable. If the offset option is not declared, the estimated coefficients will be different because there will not be an adjustment for the population size.

10.7 Definition of Adjusted Relative Risk

When the exposure E is a dichotomous variable coded as 1 to denote the presence of the factor and 0 to denote the absence of the factor, the incidence in the exposed group using the Poisson model is estimated by the following expression:

a) Incidence in the exposed group $(E=1)$:

$$I_1 = \frac{\mu_1}{P_1} = e^{\beta_0 + \beta_E + \sum_{j=1}^{J} \beta_j C_j}$$

b) Incidence in the unexposed group $(E=0)$:

$$I_0 = \frac{\mu_0}{P_0} = e^{\beta_0 + \sum_{j=1}^{J} \beta_j C_j'}$$

Therefore, the relative risk (RR) is given by

$$RR = \frac{I_1}{I_0} = e^{\beta_E + \sum_{j=1}^{J} \beta_j \left(C_j - C_j' \right)}$$

The resulting RR expression will be the same in both types of incidences (density and cumulative) under the Poisson regression model; however, the coefficients might be different. The expression $\left(C_j - C_j' \right)$ indicates the difference in the value of the jth confounding variable between the exposed and unexposed groups. The adjusted relative risk is obtained under the assumption $C_j = C_j'$. The result of this assumption leads to the following expression:

$$RR_{adjusted} = e^{\beta_E} \tag{10.11}$$

The relative risk adjusted for the potential confounders is used to obtain a comparison between the exposed group and the unexposed group under the assumption that the confounding variables have the same value; for example, same age, same sex, and same occupation given that age, sex, and occupation are considered as confounding variables. This expression is similar to the RR_{crude} ($RR_{crude} = e^{\beta_E^*}$), which is obtained in the Poisson regression model when the only predictor is the exposure variable, while $RR_{adjusted}$ is obtained in the same model but with more than one predictor (exposure with at least one confounding variable).

10.8 Interaction Assessment

To estimate the adjusted relative risk using a Poisson regression model, it is necessary to verify that there are no interactions between the exposure and potential confounding variables. If any significant interaction terms are found, the relative risk will depend on the coefficient associated with the interaction term. For example, assuming a study that investigates a dichotomous exposure (E) and one dichotomous confounder (C) (both variables coded as 1 to denote presence and 0 to denote absence), the resulting Poisson model with the interaction term (γ) is as follows:

$$I_i = \frac{\mu_i}{P_i} = e^{\beta_0 + \beta_E E + \beta_C C + \gamma(EC)} \tag{10.12}$$

The incidence for each exposure level will be as follows:

a) Incidence in the exposed group $(E=1)$:

$$I_1 = \frac{\mu_1}{P_1} = e^{\beta_0 + \beta_E + \beta_C C + \gamma C}$$

b) Incidence in the unexposed group $(E=0)$:

$$I_0 = \frac{\mu_0}{P_0} = e^{\beta_0 + \beta_C C'}$$

As a consequence, the relative risk (exposed versus unexposed) will be as follows:

$$RR = \frac{I_1}{I_0} = e^{\beta_E + \beta_C(C-C') + \gamma C} \tag{10.13}$$

where γ represents the coefficient associated with the interaction between the exposure variable and potential confounding variable (EC). If we assume that $C = C'$, the resulting relative risk is the exponential of the coefficient associated with the exposure plus the value of the confounding variable multiplied by the coefficient γ:

$$RR = e^{\beta_E + \gamma^* C}$$

Therefore, the presence of interaction terms in the model impedes obtaining the adjusted relative risk. So, for each value of the confounder (C), an RR is computed. When $C=1$, $RR = e^{\beta_E + \gamma}$; when $C=0$, $RR = e^{\beta_E}$.

10.9 Relative Risk Estimation

The procedure for estimating the RR (crude or adjusted) using a confidence interval varies depending on how the exposure is defined. When the exposure is dichotomous (1 denotes presence and 0 denotes absence), the confidence interval is given by the following expression:

$$RR \in \left[e^{\hat{\beta}_E - Z_{1-\alpha/2}{}^* \mathrm{se}(\hat{\beta}_E)}, \ e^{\hat{\beta}_E + Z_{1-\alpha/2}{}^* \mathrm{se}(\hat{\beta}_E)} \right] \tag{10.14}$$

where

$\hat{\beta}_E$ indicates the estimated value of the coefficient associated with the exposure.

$se(\hat{\beta}_E)$ indicates the standard error of $\hat{\beta}_E$.

$Z_{1-\alpha/2}$ indicates the $1 - \alpha/2$ percentile of the standardized normal distribution.

When E is a quantitative variable, the confidence interval is given by the following expression:

$$RR \in \left[e^{\left(\hat{\beta}_E - Z_{1-(\alpha/2)}{}^* se(\hat{\beta}_E)\right){}^*\delta}, \; e^{\left(\hat{\beta}_E + Z_{1-(\alpha/2)}{}^* se(\hat{\beta}_E)\right){}^*\delta} \right]$$

where

δ indicates the difference between the two values of the exposure variable being compared. For example, if the exposure variable is the number of cigarettes smoked daily by one person, an interpretation of $\delta = 10$ may indicate the comparison of the risk of smoking 25 cigarettes versus the risk of smoking 15 cigarettes. An alternative interpretation for $\delta = 10$ is to compare the risk associated with smoking 15 cigarettes against the risk associated with smoking 5 cigarettes.

When the exposure variable is a categorical variable with K levels and we are interested in comparing the kth level versus the first level (reference category), the confidence interval is given by the following expression:

$$RR_{k \text{ versus } 1} \in \left[e^{\hat{\beta}_{E_k} - Z_{1-\alpha/2}{}^* se\left(\hat{\beta}_{E_k}\right)}, \; e^{\hat{\beta}_{E_k} + Z_{1-\alpha/2}{}^* se\left(\hat{\beta}_{E_k}\right)} \right] \tag{10.15}$$

where

$\hat{\beta}_{E_k}$ indicates the estimated effect of the kth level of the exposure variable with respect to a reference group. Usually, the reference group is defined as the category with the lowest code.

10.10 Implementation of the Poisson Regression Model

To illustrate the use of the Poisson regression model, a comparison of the incidence of non-melanoma skin cancer between the cities of Minneapolis, St. Paul, and Dallas, Fort Worth adjusting for age is presented (see Table 10.5).

Table 10.5 Incidence of non-melanoma skin cancer in Minneapolis–St. Paul and Dallas–Fort Worth.

Age group (years)	Minneapolis, St. Paul		Dallas, Fort Worth		RR[a]
	Cases	Population	Cases	Population	
15–24	1	172,675	4	181,343	3.81
25–34	16	123,065	38	146,207	2.00
35–44	30	96,216	119	121,207	3.14
45–54	71	92,051	221	111,353	2.57
55–64	102	72,159	259	83,004	2.21
65–74	130	54,722	310	55,932	2.33
75–84	133	32,185	226	29,007	1.89
≥85	40	8,328	65	7,538	1.80

a) Relative risk using Minneapolis, St. Paul as the reference city.
Source: Kleinbaum et al. (2014).

To evaluate the association between city of residence and incidence of non-melanoma skin cancer while controlling for age, the data were coded as follows:

Age group
    1 = 15–24 years
    2 = 25–34 years
    3 = 35–44 years
    4 = 45–54 years
    5 = 55–64 years
    6 = 65–74 years
    7 = 75–84 years
    8 = ≥85 years
City
    1 = Dallas–Fort Worth
    0 = Minneapolis
Cases = Number of people diagnosed with non-melanoma skin cancer
Pop = Estimated population at midyear

Therefore, the database of this study was defined as follows:

Age	City	Cases	Pop
1	0	1	172675
1	1	4	181343
2	0	16	123065

Age	City	Cases	Pop
2	1	38	146207
3	0	30	96216
3	1	119	121207
4	0	71	92051
4	1	221	111353
5	0	102	72159
5	1	259	83004
6	0	130	54722
6	1	310	55932
7	0	133	32185
7	1	226	29007
8	0	40	8328
8	1	65	7538

For the Poisson regression model, we used the *glm* command in STATA. Initially, we assessed the significance of the interaction term formed with the product of age group and city, where both variables are declared as categorical variables. We fitted the model with the interaction terms (see Table 10.6), and then fitted a second model without the interaction terms (see Table 10.7) in order to compare the *deviances* of each model using the likelihood ratio test (see Table 10.8).

The result of the *likelihood ratio test* suggested elimination of the interaction term in the Poisson regression model because it was not significant (p-value $= 0.314$). The resulting equation model without interaction terms is

$$I_i = e^{-11.7+.8^*City+2.6^*Age_2+3.9^*Age_3+4.6^*Age_4+5.1^*Age_5+5.7^*Age_6+6.1^*Age_7+6.2^*Age_8}$$

where

  City $=$ 1 if the city is Dallas, Fort Worth, 0 if the city is Minneapolis, St. Paul
  Age$_i$ $=$ 1 if the cases belong to the age group i, 0 otherwise.

It should also be noted that the model that excludes the interaction term does not show *overdispersion* problems, since the *deviance* is not far from its corresponding degrees of freedom (Deviance/df $= 1.17$).

On the basis of the model that excludes the interaction term, we evaluated the presence of confounding variables by comparing the relative risk obtained in the crude model, which contains the variable city, and the relative risk of the model

Table 10.6 Poisson model with interaction terms.

```
xi: glm cases i.city*i.age, fam(poisson) lnoff(pop) nolog
```

Generalized linear models		No. of obs	=	16
Optimization : ML		Residual df	=	0
		Scale parameter	=	1
Deviance = 1.57652e-14		(1/df) Deviance	=	.
Pearson = 1.13062e-21		(1/df) Pearson	=	.

Variance function: V(u) = u	[Poisson]	
Link function : g(u) = ln(u)	[Log]	
	AIC	= 7.890319
Log likelihood = -47.12255278	BIC	= 1.58e-14

Cases	Coefficient	OIM Std. error	z	P > |z|	95% Confidence interval	
_Icity_1	1.34	1.12	1.2	0.232	−0.85	3.53
_Iage_2	3.11	1.03	3.02	0.003	1.09	5.13
_Iage_3	3.99	1.02	3.92	0	1.99	5.98
_Iage_4	4.89	1.01	4.86	0	2.92	6.87
_Iage_5	5.50	1.00	5.47	0	3.53	7.47
_Iage_6	6.02	1.00	5.99	0	4.05	7.98
_Iage_7	6.57	1.00	6.55	0	4.60	8.54
_Iage_8	6.72	1.01	6.64	0	4.74	8.70
_IcitXage_1_2	−0.64	1.16	−0.56	0.577	−2.91	1.62
_IcitXage_1_3	−0.19	1.14	−0.17	0.867	−2.42	2.04
_IcitXage_1_4	−0.39	1.13	−0.35	0.728	−2.60	1.82
_IcitXage_1_5	−0.55	1.12	−0.49	0.628	−2.75	1.66
_IcitXage_1_6	−0.49	1.12	−0.44	0.662	−2.69	1.71
_IcitXage_1_7	−0.70	1.12	−0.63	0.531	−2.90	1.50
_IcitXage_1_8	−0.75	1.14	−0.66	0.508	−2.98	1.47
_cons	−12.06	1.00	−12.06	0	−14.02	−10.10
ln(pop)	1	(exposure)				

Table 10.7 Poisson model without interaction terms.

```
. xi: glm cases i.city i.age, fam(poisson) lnoff(pop) nolog
```

Generalized linear models		No. of obs	=	16
Optimization	: ML	Residual df	=	7
		Scale parameter	=	1
Deviance	= 8.219912208	(1/df) Deviance	=	1.174273
Pearson	= 8.085982518	(1/df) Pearson	=	1.15514
Variance function: V(u) = u		[Poisson]		
Link function	: g(u) = ln(u)	[Log]		
		AIC		= 7.529064
Log likelihood = -51.23250889		BIC		= -11.18821

Cases	Coefficient	OIM Std. error	z	P > |z|	95% Confidence interval	
_Icity_1	0.80	0.052	15.41	0.00	0.70	0.91
_Iage_2	2.63	0.467	5.63	0.00	1.71	3.55
_Iage_3	3.85	0.455	8.46	0.00	2.96	4.74
_Iage_4	4.60	0.451	10.19	0.00	3.71	5.48
_Iage_5	5.09	0.450	11.3	0.00	4.20	5.97
_Iage_6	5.65	0.450	12.55	0.00	4.76	6.53
_Iage_7	6.06	0.450	13.45	0.00	5.18	6.94
_Iage_8	6.18	0.458	13.5	0.00	5.28	7.08
_cons	−11.66	0.449	−25.98	0.00	−12.54	−10.78
ln(pop)	1.00	(exposure)				

that includes the variables city and age group. If there is a difference between the point estimates of the RR (crude versus age-adjusted), it suggests that age is a confounding variable. Tables 10.9 and 10.10 describe the estimated RRs of these models.

Table 10.8 Likelihood ratio test.

Comparison of the *log-likelihoods*:
LR chi2(7) = 8.22 = −2*(−51.23 + 47.12)
Prob > chi2 = 0.314

Table 10.9 Poisson model excluding the variable age.

```
xi: glm cases i.city , fam(poisson) lnoff(pop) nolog
noheader ef
```

Cases	IRR	OIM Std. error	z	P > |z|	95% Confidence interval	
_Icity_1	2.10	0.110	14.26	0.00	1.90	2.33
_cons	0.0008	0.00004	−163.00	0.00	0.00073	0.00087
ln(pop)	1.00	(exposure)				

Interpretation: The estimated risk of developing non-melanoma skin cancer in Dallas, Fort Worth is 2.1 (95% CI: 1.9, 2.3) times the estimated risk of developing this cancer in Minneapolis, St. Paul. This excess in risk was statistically significant (p-value <0.05).

When the relative risks of the crude and adjusted models are compared, differences in the point estimates are noted:

$$\widehat{RR}_{Crude} = 2.1 \neq \widehat{RR}_{Adjusted\ for\ age} = 2.23$$

Table 10.10 Poisson model including the variable age.

```
xi: glm cases i.city i.age, fam(poisson) lnoff(pop)
nolog noheader ef
```

Cases	IRR	OIM Std. error	z	P > |z|	95% Confidence interval	
_Icity_1	2.2	0.1	15.4	0.000	2.02	2.48
_Iage_2	13.9	6.5	5.6	0.000	5.55	34.69
_Iage_3	46.9	21.3	8.5	0.000	19.24	114.37
_Iage_4	99.0	44.7	10.2	0.000	40.90	239.65
_Iage_5	161.9	72.9	11.3	0.000	67.00	391.45
_Iage_6	283.0	127.3	12.6	0.000	117.21	683.28
_Iage_7	427.8	192.6	13.5	0.000	176.96	1033.97
_Iage_8	482.1	220.7	13.5	0.000	196.57	1182.45
_cons	8.65e-06	3.88e-06	−25.98	0.000	3.59E-06	0.00
ln(pop)	1.00	(exposure)				

Interpretation: The estimated risk of developing non-melanoma skin cancer in Dallas, Fort Worth is 2.2 (95% CI: 2.0, 2.5) times the estimated risk of developing this cancer in Minneapolis, St. Paul, adjusting for age. This excess in risk was statistically significant (p-value <0.05).

This result indicates that the RR_{crude} underestimates the magnitude of association of interest. This evaluation is subjective, as it does not involve the use of statistical tests of the observed difference. Some have argued that confounding can be considered to be present if the estimates of the crude and adjusted relative risks differ by at least 10% (Rothman et al., 2008). Although this rule of thumb provides a simple and easily applicable method to identify confounders, the conceptual framework and current state of knowledge of association under investigation should guide the model building process (Bliss et al., 2012).

When we observe the RRs presented in Table 10.5, the results suggest that age is an effect modifier in the association between city of residence and the risk of developing non-melanoma skin cancer, even though there were no significant interaction terms in the Poisson regression model (p-value >0.05). As a consequence, we may be interested in assessing the RR of each age group, after running the model with interaction terms (see Table 10.6). The following are the STATA outputs to estimate the RR between cities for each age group using the *lincom* command after running the Poisson model with interaction terms:

```
*For age-group 15-24 years
. lincom _Icity_1,  rr
 ( 1)  [cases]_Icity_1 = 0
```

Cases	IRR	Std. error	z	P > |z|	95% Confidence interval	
(1)	3.8	4.26	1.20	0.23	0.43	34.08

Interpretation: Among subjects aged 15–24 years, the risk of developing non-melanoma skin cancer in Dallas, Fort Worth is 3.8 (95% CI: 0.4, 34.1) times the risk of developing this cancer in Minneapolis, St. Paul. However, this excess was not statistically significant (p-value >0.05).

```
*For age-group 25-34 years
. lincom _Icity_1 +  _IcitXage_1_2,  rr
 ( 1)  [cases]_Icity_1 + [cases]_IcitXage_1_2 = 0
```

Cases	IRR	Std. error	z	P > |z|	95% Confidence interval	
(1)	2.0	0.60	2.32	0.02	1.11	3.59

Interpretation: Among subjects aged 25–34 years, the estimated risk of developing non-melanoma skin cancer in Dallas, Fort Worth is 2.0 (95% CI: 1.1, 3.6) times the risk of developing this cancer in Minneapolis, St. Paul. This excess was statistically significant (p-value <0.05).

```
*For age-group 35-44 years
. lincom _Icity_1 +  _IcitXage_1_3,   rr
 ( 1)  [cases]_Icity_1 + [cases]_IcitXage_1_3 = 0
```

Cases	IRR	Std. error	z	P > |z|	95% Confidence interval	
(1)	3.2	0.64	5.61	0.000	2.11	4.70

Interpretation: Among subjects aged 35–44 years, the estimated risk of developing non-melanoma skin cancer in Dallas, Fort Worth is 3.2 (95% CI: 2.1, 4.7) times the risk of developing this cancer in Minneapolis, St. Paul. This excess was statistically significant (p-value <0.05).

```
*For age-group 45-54 years
. lincom _Icity_1 +  _IcitXage_1_4,   rr
 ( 1)  [cases]_Icity_1 + [cases]_IcitXage_1_4 = 0
```

Cases	IRR	Std. error	z	P > |z|	95% Confidence interval	
(1)	2.6	0.35	6.93	0.000	1.97	3.36

Interpretation: Among subjects aged 45–54 years, the estimated risk of developing non-melanoma skin cancer in Dallas, Fort Worth is 2.6 (95% CI: 2.0, 3.4) times the risk of developing this cancer in Minneapolis, St. Paul. This excess was statistically significant (p-value <0.05).

```
*For age-group 55-64 years
. lincom _Icity_1 +  _IcitXage_1_5,   rr
 ( 1)  [cases]_Icity_1 + [cases]_IcitXage_1_5 = 0
```

Cases	IRR	Std. error	z	P > |z|	95% Confidence interval	
(1)	2.2	0.26	6.77	0.000	1.76	2.78

Interpretation: Among subjects aged 55–64 years, the estimated risk of developing non-melanoma skin cancer in Dallas, Fort Worth is 2.2 (95% CI: 1.8, 2.8) times the risk of developing this cancer in Minneapolis, St. Paul. This excess was statistically significant (p-value <0.05).

```
*For age-group 65-74 years
. lincom _Icity_1 +  _IcitXage_1_6,  rr
  ( 1)  [cases]_Icity_1 + [cases]_IcitXage_1_6 = 0
```

Cases	IRR	Std. error	z	P > |z|	95% Confidence interval	
(1)	2.3	0.24	8.11	0.000	1.90	2.86

Interpretation: Among subjects aged 65–74 years, the estimated risk of developing non-melanoma skin cancer in Dallas, Fort Worth is 2.3 (95% CI: 1.9, 2.9) times the risk of developing this cancer in Minneapolis, St. Paul. This excess was statistically significant (p-value <0.05).

```
*For age-group 75-84 years
. lincom _Icity_1 +  _IcitXage_1_7,  rr
  ( 1)  [cases]_Icity_1 + [cases]_IcitXage_1_7 = 0
```

Cases	IRR	Std. error	z	P > |z|	95% Confidence interval	
(1)	1.9	0.21	5.80	0.000	1.52	2.34

Interpretation: Among subjects aged 75–84 years, the estimated risk of developing non-melanoma skin cancer in Dallas, Fort Worth is 1.9 (95% CI: 1.5, 2.3) times the risk of developing this cancer in Minneapolis, St. Paul. This excess was statistically significant (p-value <0.05).

```
*For age-group 85 years or more
. lincom _Icity_1 +  _IcitXage_1_8,  rr
  ( 1)  [cases]_Icity_1 + [cases]_IcitXage_1_8 = 0
```

Cases	IRR	Std. error	z	P > |z|	95% Confidence interval	
(1)	1.8	0.36	2.91	0.000	1.21	2.66

Interpretation: Among subjects aged 85 years or more, the estimated risk of developing non-melanoma skin cancer in Dallas, Fort Worth is 1.8 (95% CI: 1.2, 2.7) times the risk of developing this cancer in Minneapolis, St. Paul. This excess was statistically significant (*p*-value <0.05).

All groups show a significant increment in the risk of developing non-melanoma skin cancer in Dallas, Fort Worth (*p*-value <0.05), with the only exception in the subjects between 15–24 years old.

10.11 Conclusion

The procedure to assess the magnitude of the association of interest in a Poisson regression model involves a careful assessment of confounding variables and effect modification. Several approaches are available to building a regression model for assessing the significance of the relationship between exposure and disease (Gerstman, 1998; Szklo and Nieto, 2007; Rothman et al, 2008). The main concern is the subjectivity in assessing the confounding effect, when comparing the point estimates of the crude RR and adjusted RR. How large should this difference be? Recent recommendations for declaring no confounding effect is to keep the ratio between $\hat{RR}_{adjusted}$ and $\hat{RR}_{crude}$ within the following range: $0.9 < (\hat{RR}_{adjusted}/\hat{RR}_{crude}) < 1.1$ (Greenland et al., 2016). The other concern is the assessment of effect modification by confounding variables: Should this assessment be performed before or after a regression model without interaction terms is built? The evaluation of effect modification is important for determining how to carry out the statistical analysis. The *Mantel–Haenszel* method and the Poisson model allow us to formally assess the presence of interaction. However, some inconsistencies might be seen when stratum-specific RRs are compared, the RRs could be very different when no significant interaction terms are shown in the Poisson model. This could be explained by the sample size in each stratum, after stratifying the study group, particularly when the incidence of the disease of interest is low. Our recommendation is to collapse stratums, if possible, before exploring the magnitude of the association of interest. If there is no evidence of interaction terms in the model, then estimate the adjusted RR and declare whether or not the results were significant. However, the implementation of any statistical analysis is always complicated by problems associated with small sample size, complex interrelationships among the variable under consideration, and the inherent limitations of the statistical procedures used. Indeed, the ability to carry out a well-conceived multivariate analysis of a complex epidemiologic data set requires an in-depth theoretical understanding of the statistical procedures involved and an appreciation of the disease etiology as a function of the disease of interest. Such analyses are best carried out in an interactive environment that includes both biostatisticians and epidemiologists (Kleinbaum *et al.*, 1982).

Practice Exercise

The following table summarizes the data of a cohort study designed to test the hypothesis that obesity increases the risk of cardiovascular disease (CVD):

Age in years	Obese status	CVD	Person-years
60–64	Obese	10	245
	Not obese	12	640
65–69	Obese	34	365
	Not obese	45	520
70–74	Obese	40	250
	Not obese	44	490

a) Evaluate the significance of the interaction between age and obesity using a Poisson regression model.

b) Estimate the relative risk of CVD according to obesity using a 95% confidence interval.

c) Estimate the relative risk of CVD according to obesity for each age group using a 95% confidence interval.

d) Estimate the relative risk of CVD according to obesity status adjusting for age group using a 95% confidence interval.

References

Bliss, R., Weinberg, J., Webster, T., and Vieira, V. (2012) Determining the probability distribution and evaluating sensitivity and false positive rate of a confounder detection method applied to logistic regression. *J. Biom. Biostat.*, **3**, 142.

Gerstman, B. (1998) *Epidemiology Kept Simple: An Introduction to Classic and Modern Epidemiology*. New York: John Wiley & Sons, Inc.

Gordis, L. (2014) *Epidemiology*, 5th edition. Philadelphia, PA: Elsevier Saunders.

Greenland, S., Daniel, R., and Pearce, N. (2016) Outcome modelling strategies in epidemiology: traditional methods and basic alternatives. *Int. J. Epidemiol.*, **45**, 1–11.

Jewell, N. (2004) *Statistics for Epidemiology*. Boca Raton, FL: Chapman & Hall/ CRC.

Kleinbaum, D.G., Kupper, L.L., and Morgenstern, H. (1982) *Epidemiologic Research: Principles and Quantitative Methods*. New York: John Wiley & Sons, Inc.

Kleinbaum, D.G., Kupper, L.L., Nizam, A., and Rosenberg, E.S. (2014) *Applied Regression Analysis and Other Multivariable Methods*, 5th edition. Boston, MA: Cengage Learning.

Rosner, B. (2010) *Fundamentals of Biostatistics*, 7th edition. Boston, MA: Cengage Learning.

Rothman, K.J., Greenland, S., and Lash, T.L. (2012) *Modern Epidemiology*, 3rd edition. Philadelphia, PA: Lippincott Williams & Wilkins.

Selvin, S. (2004) *Statistical Analysis of Epidemiologic Data*, 3rd edition. New York, NY: Oxford University Press.

Szklo, M. and Nieto, F.J. (2007) *Epidemiology Beyond the Basics*, 2nd edition. Sudbury, MA: Jones and Bartlett.

VanderWeele, T.J. (2009) On the distinction between interaction and effect modification. *Epidemiology*, **20**, 863–871.

11

Logistic Regression in Case–Control Studies

Aim: Upon completing this chapter, the reader should be able to fit a generalized linear model for binary and binomial responses in case–control study designs.

11.1 Introduction

This chapter presents the analytical strategies to evaluate the data obtained from a *case–control* study design. The purpose of this design is to assess the magnitude of the association between an exposure and a specific disease or health-related event. The simplest design for a case–control study is composed of two groups of subjects: (i) subjects newly diagnosed with the disease of interest, called *cases*, and (ii) subjects without the disease of interest, called *controls*. Once these are identified, we measure and compare the prevalence of exposure to a certain factor in the two groups. This is the most cost-effective analytical epidemiological study design and is recommended when the incidence of the disease or condition of interest is low or has a long latency period (Gordis, 2014).

The sampling procedures for selecting subjects for a case–control design could be based on the setting the cases are selected from, regardless of the population from which they arise (i.e., population based, hospital based, clinic based, or community based). Control participants must be identical to case participants, except that they do not have the disease, and they should be drawn from the same population from which the cases arise. However, sometimes cases and controls are selected from different data sources. For example, cases may be selected from a disease registry but the controls are selected randomly from the population. Because controls are used to estimate the distribution of exposure in the source population, the basic requirement of control selection is that the controls be sampled independent of exposure status.

Applications of Regression Models in Epidemiology, First Edition. Erick Suárez,
Cynthia M. Pérez, Roberto Rivera, and Melissa N. Martínez.
© 2017 John Wiley & Sons, Inc. Published 2017 by John Wiley & Sons, Inc.

Matching is an option that can improve efficiency in the comparison between cases and controls by protecting against the situation where the distribution of confounding variables differs substantially between them (Wacholder et al., 1992a, 1992b, 1992c; 1995). The matching procedure could be based on individual matching or frequency matching. In an individually matched case–control study, each case is matched to one or more controls based on one or more variables (i.e., same age or same sex) that are defined *a priori* as potential confounders. In frequency matching, a group of cases is matched to a group of controls, keeping a balanced number of cases and controls across the strata defined by the potential confounders. While matching is intended to eliminate confounding variables, the main potential benefit of matching in case–control studies is a gain in efficiency. Without matching, control for confounding in the analysis will result in many strata with sparse data. By balancing the distribution of cases and controls across strata, the estimates of the magnitude of the association of interest will be more stable—smaller standard errors, and thus narrower confidence intervals. However, overmatching could be counterproductive if the matching variables are closely related with the exposure to be evaluated, causing the magnitude of the association to be biased toward the null hypothesis, H_0: OR $= 1$ (Rothman et al., 2012).

11.2 Specific Objectives

- Define the concepts of crude and adjusted odds ratios (ORs) to assess the magnitude of the association between an exposure and a specific disease using a logistic regression model.
- Assess confounding and effect modification using the results of the logistic regression model.

11.3 Graphical Representation

A basic way to represent an unmatched case–control study design is depicted in Figure 11.1.

To assess disease risk during a certain time in a specific population, one statistical measure used is the incidence of the disease. Having established the impact on different groups of exposure, it is possible to estimate the magnitude of the association through the relative risk (incidence in the exposed group/ incidence of unexposed group). However, in a case–control study it is not possible to compute incidence of disease because the study subjects are selected based on their disease status (cases or controls). Therefore, to assess the magnitude of the association between exposure and disease, the *odds ratio* is computed.

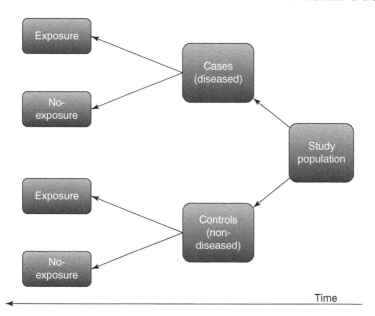

Figure 11.1 Basic design of an unmatched case–control study design.

11.4 Definition of the Odds Ratio

In an unmatched case–control study design, it is not possible to directly estimate disease incidence in those who are exposed and those who are unexposed, since participants are selected according to the disease status, not on the basis of their exposure status. However, it is possible to calculate the odds of exposure among cases and controls, as follows:

- *Odds* of exposure among cases = Expected number of exposed for each non-exposed among cases:

$$= \frac{P_{\text{exposed cases}}}{1 - P_{\text{exposed cases}}} = \frac{\text{Probability of exposure among cases}}{\text{Probability of non-exposure among cases}} \quad (11.1)$$

- *Odds* of exposure among controls = Expected number of exposed for each non-exposed among controls:

$$= \frac{P_{\text{exposed controls}}}{1 - P_{\text{exposed controls}}} = \frac{\text{Probability of exposure among controls}}{\text{Probability of non-exposure among controls}}$$

$$(11.2)$$

- P_i indicates the probability of being exposed in the ith group (cases or controls).

The exposure odds ratio is defined as the ratio of the odds of the exposure in cases to that in controls, as follows:

$$OR_{exposure} = \frac{Odds_{exposure\ in\ cases}}{Odds_{exposure\ in\ controls}} \tag{11.3}$$

It can be shown algebraically that the $OR_{exposure}$ obtained from a case–control study provides an analogous expression for the disease odds ratio, as follows:

$$OR_{disease} = \frac{Odds_{disease\ among\ exposed}}{Odds_{disease\ among\ unexposed}} \tag{11.4}$$

where

- $Odds_{disease\ among\ exposed}$ indicates the expected number of cases for each control in the exposed group.
- $Odds_{disease\ among\ unexposed}$ indicates the expected number of cases for each control in the unexposed group.

11.5 Confounding Assessment

To evaluate the effect of potential confounding variables in a case–control study, it is necessary to compare the point estimate of the crude odds ratio $\left(\widehat{OR}_{crude}\right)$ and the point estimate of the adjusted odds ratio $(\widehat{OR}_{adjusted})$. This is a subjective comparison of the point estimate as there is not a formal statistical test to assess the presence of confounding. In general, if the $\widehat{OR}_{crude}$ is similar to $\widehat{OR}_{adjusted}$, it is concluded that the confounding variables have no effect in the magnitude of the association of interest. Otherwise, it is recommended to determine if the $\widehat{OR}_{crude}$ overestimates or underestimates the association of interest using as a reference the $\widehat{OR}_{adjusted}$.

11.6 Effect Modification

When the magnitude of the association between the exposure and disease does not behave the same way across the levels of a third variable, that is, there is no homogeneity among the ORs, it is said that there is effect modification. For example, assume that the values of ORs for the association between diabetes (exposure) and cardiovascular disease (outcome) in males and females are described in Table 11.1.

Table 11.1 Example of the magnitude of the association between diabetes and cardiovascular disease by sex.

Sex (stratum)	OR$_{\text{Diabetes + versus Diabetes –}}$
Females	2.2
Males	6.3
Both groups	4.3

Based on visual inspection of the data in Table 11.1, the magnitude of the association between diabetes and cardiovascular disease is different across strata, suggesting the presence of effect modification. In this example, the OR in females is 2.2 and the OR in males is 6.3. When there is effect modification (no homogeneity of the ORs), it is advisable to assess the magnitude of the association of interest in each stratum. Evaluation of the overall effect of the confounding variable, if effect modification is present, would obscure the relationship between exposure and disease (Szklo and Nieto, 2007).

11.7 Stratified Analysis

In a case–control study it is also recommended to assess the association in different strata defined by levels of the confounding variables. For each stratum, an OR$_k$ is estimated for the association of interest in order to assess effect modification. As we described in the previous chapter, the *Mantel–Haenszel* method has been used to test the homogeneity of the ORs over different strata when the exposure is categorized in two groups. This method uses the following estimate of a common OR, which is valid when the ORs in each stratum are homogeneous (absence of effect modification):

$$\text{OR}_{\text{MH}} = \sum_{k=1}^{K} \frac{w_k \text{OR}_k}{w_k} \tag{11.5}$$

where w_k is the weighted factor in the kth stratum, which is determined as the product of the number of cases that are unexposed and the number of controls that are exposed divided by the number of subjects in this stratum. An example of an unmatched case–control study is described in Table 11.2, which aimed to assess the relationship between chronic kidney disease

Table 11.2 Chronic kidney disease (CKD) by anemia status, hypertension (HTN), and diabetes mellitus (DM): an example of unmatched case–control study.

		CKD			
Group	Anemia	Present	Absent	$\widehat{OR}$	M-H Weight
HTN-, DM-	Normal	1217	2285	Reference	37.94
	Abnormal	165	118	2.63	
HTN+, DM-	Normal	1674	1431	Reference	18.67
	Abnormal	352	39	7.72	
HTN-, DM+	Normal	383	588	Reference	5.62
	Abnormal	36	15	3.68	
HTN+, DM+	Normal	1189	634	Reference	13.77
	Abnormal	310	25	6.61	
Overall	Normal	4463	4938	Reference	
	Abnormal	863	197	4.85	

Source: Sui-Lung et al. (2015).

(CKD) and anemia, controlling for hypertension (HTN) and diabetes mellitus (DM).

The point estimates of the ORs in each group in Table 11.2 show large differences between them, especially when the group is composed of subjects with hypertension, which suggests that the combination of hypertension and diabetes could be an effect modifier in the association between anemia and CKD. A formal assessment of effect modification will be discussed in the section 11.13 using a logistic regression model. Assuming that absence of effect modification is justified, the point estimate of the common OR, using *Mantel–Haenszel* method, is $\widehat{OR}_{MH} = 4.67$. Then, the comparison of $\widehat{OR}_{MH} = 4.67$ with $\widehat{OR}_{Crude} = 4.85$ would suggest the presence of confounding and that the OR_{crude} could overestimate the magnitude of association.

11.8 Unconditional Logistic Regression Model

One of the generalized linear models most used in epidemiological studies is the logistic regression model. This model allows us to estimate the OR (crude and adjusted) to assess the magnitude of the association between the exposure of interest and the disease under study. For example, in an unmatched case–control study to estimate the OR, we need to estimate the probability of having the disease in the exposed and unexposed groups and calculate the OR as follows:

$$OR = \frac{P_{\text{exposed}}/(1 - P_{\text{exposed}})}{P_{\text{unexposed}}/(1 - P_{\text{unexposed}})} \tag{11.6}$$

To estimate these probabilities under different conditions, we can use the unconditional logistic regression (ULR) model in an unmatched case–control study, as follows:

$$p_i = \frac{1}{1 + e^{-(\beta_0 + \beta_E E_i + \Sigma_{j=1}^{J} \beta_j C_{i,j})}} \tag{11.7}$$

where

p_i: indicates the probability of having the disease under the conditions i. These conditions i indicate a combination of the values of the predictor variables (including exposure and of confounding variables).

E_i: indicates the exposure factor under study under the condition i. This variable can be quantitative or categorical. In the case of a dichotomous variable we can define an indicator variable (*dummy variable*) such as 1 if the exposure factor is present and 0 if absent.

$C_{i,j}$: indicates a potential confounding variable under the condition i, for $j = 1, \ldots, m$.

β_E: indicates the coefficient associated with the exposure.

β_j: indicates the coefficient associated with each jth confounding variable.

Therefore, the probability of observing a control (nondiseased person) through the ULR model is

$$1 - p_i = 1 - \frac{1}{1 + e^{-(\beta_0 + \beta_E E_i + \Sigma_{j=1}^{J} \beta_j C_{i,j})}} \tag{11.8}$$

As a result, the odds of disease can be defined by

$$\frac{p_i}{1 - p_i} = e^{(\beta_0 + \beta_E E_i + \Sigma_{j=1}^{J} \beta_j C_{i,j})} \tag{11.9}$$

On a logarithmic scale, the odds of disease would be

$$\ln\left(\frac{p_i}{1 - p_i}\right) = \beta_0 + \beta_E E_i + \Sigma_{j=1}^{J} \beta_j C_{i,j} \tag{11.10}$$

where $\ln(p_i/(1 - p_i))$ is defined as the *logit function* or *logit* p_i.

11.9 Types of Logistic Regression Models

Depending on the way information is collected, the ULR model applies in two scenarios to assess the likelihood of becoming ill: the binary case and the binomial case.

Table 11.3 Example data for ULR model: binary case.

Confounding variables		Exposure	Case/Control
C_1	C_2	E	Y
30	1	1	0
12	1	0	1
43	0	1	1
⋮	⋮	⋮	⋮

11.9.1 Binary Case

The random variable under study (Y) is collected as *dichotomous* (0,1). For example, assume that Y defines the type of subject (case or control). Usually this variable is coded as $Y = 1$ to denote the person categorized as case, while $Y = 0$ is used to denote the person categorized as control. Suppose we have data from a case–control study with an exposure factor ($E = 0,1$; where 0 denotes the unexposed person while 1 denotes the exposed person) and two confounding variables (C1 and C2). The data might be as shown in Table 11.3.

In this hypothetical case, the first person is a control ($Y = 0$) who is exposed to the factor of interest ($E = 1$) and has values of 30 and 1 for the potential confounding variables C_1 and C_2. The next subject is a case ($Y = 1$) who is not exposed to the factor of interest and has values of 12 and 1 for the potential confounding variables C_1 and C_2.

11.9.2 Binomial Case

In the binomial case, the random variable under study (Y) is collected as the number of sick people from the total number observed persons. In this case we say that the data are *grouped*. The composition of the data for a binomial random variable Y with two potential confounding variables (C_1 and C_2) and the exposure factor ($E = 0,1$; where 0 denotes the unexposed person while 1 denotes the exposed person) is presented in Table 11.4.

The first row indicates that 20 exposed people ($E = 1$) were ill at the time of the study based on 250 subjects, where the confounding variables showed the following values: $C_1 = 30$ and $C_2 = 1$. The second line indicates that 30 non-exposed persons ($E = 0$) were ill at the time of study based on 55 subjects, where the confounding variables showed the following values: $C_1 = 12$ and $C_2 = 1$. And so on for the remaining rows.

Table 11.4 Data for ULR model: binomial case.

Confounding variables		Exposure	Cases	Total
C_1	C_2	E		
30	1	1	20	250
12	1	0	30	55
43	0	1	1	7
⋮	⋮	⋮	⋮	⋮

11.10 Computing the OR$_{crude}$

The process to obtain the OR$_{crude}$ in the ULR model (when the only predictor in the model is the exposure) is as follows:

1) Identify the odds in the simple ULR model. Assuming that the exposure factor is a dichotomous variable ($E=0,1$; where 0 denotes the unexposed person, while 1 denotes the exposed person), the *odds* would be
   i) *Odds* of disease in the exposed group ($E=1$)

$$\text{Odds}_1 = \frac{p_1}{1-p_1} = e^{\beta_0 + \beta_E}$$

   ii) *Odds* of disease in the unexposed group ($E=0$)

$$\text{Odds}_0 = \frac{p_0}{1-p_0} = e^{\beta_0}$$

2) Calculate the crude odds ratio

$$\text{OR}_{Crude} = \frac{\text{Odds}_1}{\text{Odds}_0} = e^{\beta_E}$$

11.11 Computing the Adjusted OR

The process to obtain the adjusted OR in the presence of potential confounding variables in the ULR is as follows:

i) Identify the odds in the ULR model for each exposure level. Assuming that the exposure is a dichotomous variable ($E=0,1$; where 0 denotes the unexposed person while 1 denotes the exposed person), the odds would be

a) Odds of disease in the exposed group ($E = 1$) given specific values for the confounding variable (C_j)

$$Odds_1 = \frac{p_1}{1 - p_1} = e^{\beta_0 + \beta_E + \sum_{j=1}^{J} \beta_j C_j} \tag{11.11}$$

b) Odds of disease in the unexposed group ($E = 0$) given another set of specific values for the confounding variable (C_j')

$$Odds_0 = \frac{p_0}{1 - p_0} = e^{\beta_0 + \sum_{j=1}^{J} \beta_j C_j'} \tag{11.12}$$

ii) Calculate the OR under the logistic regression model

$$OR = \frac{Odds_1}{Odds_0} = e^{\beta_E + \sum_{j=1}^{J} \beta_j (C - C_j')} \tag{11.13}$$

When the values of the confounding variables are set equal in both groups ($C_j - C_j' = 0$) and the exposure factor is dichotomous, the adjusted OR is defined by the expression: $OR_{adjusted} = e^{\beta_E}$. To ensure the validity of the $OR_{adjusted}$, it is necessary to check beforehand that there is no interaction effect between the confounding variables and the exposure factor (see section 10.8).

11.12 Inference on OR

In an unmatched case–control study, we can estimate the OR (crude or adjusted) of the population using a confidence interval of confidence level $(1 - \alpha)\%$. This varies according to the definition of the exposure factor. Below are different ways to construct the confidence interval:

i) The exposure factor is a dichotomous variable, that is, in the factor there are two possible results (presence versus absence) that are encoded by 0 (absence) and 1 (present).

$$OR \in \left(e^{\hat{\beta}_E - Z_{1-\alpha/2} \cdot se(\hat{\beta}_E)}, \ e^{\hat{\beta}_E + Z_{1-\alpha/2} \cdot se(\hat{\beta}_E)} \right) \tag{11.14}$$

ii) The exposure factor is quantitative, where specific values will be compared (i.e., subjects who smoke 20 cigarettes daily versus those who smoke 5 cigarettes daily). The difference between these values is identified by Δ.

$$OR^\Delta \in \left(e^{[\hat{\beta}_E - Z_{1-(\alpha/2)} \cdot se(\hat{\beta}_E)] \cdot \Delta}, \ e^{[\hat{\beta}_E + Z_{1-(\alpha/2)} \cdot se(\hat{\beta}_E)] \cdot \Delta} \right) \tag{11.15}$$

iii) The exposure factor is categorical with different levels, where the comparison is between one category (k) and a reference category (assuming it is the one with the lowest code).

$$OR^{k \text{ versus } 1} \in \left(e^{\hat{\theta}_k - Z_{1-\alpha/2} \cdot se(\hat{\theta}_k)}, \ e^{\hat{\theta}_k + Z_{1-(\alpha/2)} \cdot se(\hat{\theta}_k)} \right) \tag{11.16}$$

The definition of terms used in this confidence interval is as follows:

$\hat{\beta}_E$: indicates the estimated regression coefficient associated with the exposure factor under study.

$\hat{\theta}_k$: indicates the effect of the level k of exposure factor with respect to a reference level.

se: indicates the standard error.

z: indicates the percentile $(1 - (\alpha/2))$ of the standard normal distribution, which defines the confidence level $(1 - \alpha)$ of the two-sided interval. If a 95% confidence interval is desired, then $Z = 1.96$ and $\alpha = 0.05$.

Δ: indicates the difference between the two values of a quantitative exposure.

11.13 Example of the Application of ULR Model: Binomial Case

Problem

Assume that a hypothetical case–control study was performed to determine the magnitude of the association between lung cancer and cigarette smoking, controlling for age and sex. Consider that the data collected for this study are described in Table 11.5.

Table 11.5 Hypothetical data to assess the association between lung cancer and cigarette smoking by age and sex.

Sex	Age (years)	Smoke +(yes) – (no)	Cases	Controls	$\widehat{Odds}$ of disease	$\widehat{OR}$
	35–64	+	12	12	$12/12 = 1.00$	
		–	11	20	$11/20 = 0.55$	1.82
Female	65–74	+	23	23	$23/23 = 1.00$	
		–	20	30	$20/30 = 0.67$	1.50
	≥ 75	+	31	31	$31/31 = 1.00$	
		–	13	17	$13/17 = 0.76$	1.31
	35–64	+	18	12	$18/12 = 1.50$	
		–	11	13	$11/13 = 0.85$	1.77
Male	65–74	+	78	55	$78/55 = 1.42$	
		–	50	56	$50/56 = 0.89$	1.60
	≥ 75	+	35	70	$35/70 = 0.50$	
		–	25	70	$25/70 = 0.36$	1.39

To determine whether there is an association between lung cancer and cigarette smoking, the data of Table 11.5 were analyzed through a ULR model. Given that the data are grouped, the model to be used is the binomial case. We fitted the model with the interaction terms (see Table 11.6), and then fitted a second model without the interaction terms (see Table 11.7) in order to compare the *deviances* of each model using the likelihood ratio test (see Table 11.8).

This comparison of *deviances* in Table 11.8 provides evidence to eliminate the interaction terms from the logistic regression model, since these were not

Table 11.6 Model with interaction terms.

```
. gen total=cases + controls
. xi: glm cases i.smoke*i.age i.smoke*i.sex, fam(bin total)

*Output

Generalized linear models          No. of obs     =        12
Optimization    : ML               Residual df    =         4
                                   Scale parameter =        1
Deviance        =   10.15355565    (1/df) Deviance = 2.538389
Pearson         =   10.29972147    (1/df) Pearson  = 2.57493

Variance function: V(u) = u*(1-u/total)   [Binomial]
Link function    : g(u) = ln(u/(total-u)) [Logit]

                                   AIC            = 6.528334
Log likelihood  = -31.17000505     BIC            = .213929
```

Cases	Coefficient	OIM Std. error	z	P > |z|	95% Confidence interval	
_Ismoke_1	0.69	0.42	1.63	0.103	−0.139	1.511
_Iage_2	0.20	0.32	0.62	0.537	−0.436	0.836
_Iage_3	−0.42	0.35	−1.22	0.223	−1.101	0.257
_IsmoXage_1_2	−0.15	0.45	−0.32	0.748	−1.032	0.742
_IsmoXage_1_3	−0.22	0.47	−0.47	0.640	−1.139	0.700
_Isex_2	0.00	0.25	−0.01	0.991	−0.486	0.480
_IsmoXsex_1_2	−0.10	0.33	−0.31	0.756	−0.748	0.543
_cons	−0.40	0.30	−1.37	0.171	−0.983	0.175

Table 11.7 Model without interaction terms.

```
. xi: glm cases i.smoke i.age i.sex, fam(bin total) nolog

Generalized linear models                 No. of obs      =        12
Optimization      : ML                    Residual df     =         7
                                          Scale parameter =         1
Deviance       =   10.52056254            (1/df) Deviance = 1.502938
Pearson        =   10.64525708            (1/df) Pearson  = 1.520751

Variance function: V(u) = u*(1-u/total)   [Binomial]
Link function    : g(u) = ln(u/(total-u)) [Logit]

                                          AIC             = 6.058918
Log likelihood   =  -31.3535085           BIC             =-6.873784
```

Cases	Coefficient	OIM Std. error	z	P > |z|	95% Confidence interval	
_Ismoke_1	0.47	0.15	3.070	0.002	0.168	0.766
_Iage_2	0.13	0.23	0.570	0.568	−0.313	0.570
_Iage_3	−0.53	0.23	−2.300	0.021	−0.987	−0.080
_Isex_2	−0.05	0.16	−0.320	0.746	−0.370	0.265
_cons	−0.30	0.22	−1.340	0.180	−0.735	0.138

significant ($p > 0.1$). We also observe that the model without the interaction terms does not present overdispersion problems, since the *deviance* is not far from the corresponding degrees of freedom ($10.5 \sim 7$). If a significance test on overdispersion is performed using the chi-square distribution, the resulting p-value is 0.16.

Once the interaction terms of the model and problems of overdispersion are dismissed, the next stage of the statistical analysis is to evaluate the presence of confounding variables. To conduct this evaluation, first we fitted the crude

Table 11.8 Likelihood ratio test.

Model	Deviance	Degrees of freedom	Deviance difference	p-value
With interaction terms	10.15	4	–	–
Without interaction terms	10.52	7	0.37	0.9470

Table 11.9 Crude and adjusted ORs for association between lung cancer and cigarette smoking.

Cases	OR_{crude}	OIM Std. error	z	$P > \|z\|$	[95% Confidence interval]	
_Ismoke_1	1.5	0.23	2.87	0.004	1.15	2.06

Cases	$OR_{adjusted}$	OIM Std. error	z	$P > \|z\|$	[95% Confidence interval]	
_Ismoke_1	1.6	0.24	3.07	0.00	1.18	2.15
_Iage_2	1.1	0.26	0.57	0.568	0.73	1.77
_Iage_3	0.6	0.14	−2.30	0.021	0.37	0.92
_Isex_2	0.9	0.15	−0.32	0.746	0.69	1.30

model (the model containing only the exposure smoking). Then, we fitted the model with all potential confounding variables in this study (age and sex), plus the variable smoking. For each of these two models the ORs of lung cancer and smoking were estimated (see Table 11.9).

According to the observed data in Table 11.9, there is a minimal difference between the OR point estimates ($\widehat{OR}_{crude} = 1.5$ versus $\widehat{OR}_{adjusted} = 1.6$), which might suggest that there is no confounding effect. This is a subjective comparison so caution is advised in making this comparison since different researchers may reach opposite conclusions. If in doubt, you should not rule out potential confounding variables, especially if previous studies have shown that the risk factors under consideration have shown confounding effects. The interpretation of each OR is as follows:

$\widehat{OR}_{crude}$ The estimated odds of having a person diagnosed with lung cancer in the smoking group is 1.5 (95% CI: 1.15, 2.06) times the estimated odds of having a person diagnosed with lung cancer in the nonsmoking group.

$\widehat{OR}_{adjusted}$ The estimated odds of having a person diagnosed with lung cancer in the smoking group is 1.60 (95% CI: 1.18, 2.15) times the estimated *odds* of having a person diagnosed with lung cancer in the nonsmoking group, after adjusting for age and sex.

11.14 Conditional Logistic Regression Model

An alternative to adjusting for the effect of confounding variables in the ULR model is to match cases and controls for a small number of these variables in the study design. The *matched case–control study* enables this to be achieved, in which each diseased person included in the study as a case is matched to one or more disease-free persons who will be included as controls. This type of matching is called individual matching. Common matching variables are age and sex. Continuous matching variables, such as age, are matched within a prespecified range. A design with M controls per case is known as a 1:M matched study. The individuals that constitute the one case and the M controls to which the case has been matched are referred as a *matched set*. The main disadvantage of this design is the difficulty in finding suitable matches, especially when there are several matching variables. The other concern is the overmatching that occurs when the matching variables are strongly related to the exposure under study, in which case the strength of the association between exposure and disease will be closer to unity. This may simply result in loss of efficiency, and may also cause biased results (Woodward, 2014).

When a case–control study is matched, the analysis must take the matching into account. If the standard unmatched analysis is used, the odds ratio will tend to be closer to unity. This is because the cases and controls will be more similar to each other than they would have been, if unmatched case–control study had taken place. Therefore, the results should be presented in terms of the study matched sets; it means that each member of these sets is classified according to the level of exposure and is either a case or a control. The usual distribution of these matched sets provided by a matched case–control (1:1) design with dichotomous exposure is summarized in Table 11.10.

Table 11.10 Observed counts of matched pairs in a (1:1) design.

| | | Controls | |
	Exposure	Present	Absent
Cases	Present	A	B
	Absent	C	D

where

A indicates the number of pairs where cases and controls are exposed.
B indicates the number of pairs where cases are exposed and control are not.
C indicates the number of pairs where cases are unexposed and control are exposed.
D indicates the number of pairs where cases and controls are not exposed.
$A + D$ are the concordant pairs (exposure does not differ between cases and controls).
$B + C$ are the discordant pairs (exposure differs between cases and controls).

For a given discordant pair, either the case or the control has a history of exposure. Let π_k denote the probability that in the kth discordant pair the case is exposed and the control is unexposed. The Mantel–Haenszel odds ratio for a (1:1) matched case–control study in the kth matched set is defined as follows (Newman, 2001):

$$OR_k = \frac{\pi_k}{1 - \pi_k} \tag{11.17}$$

Assuming that π_k is constant for all matched set of individuals, the estimate of π is as follows:

$$\hat{\pi} = \frac{B}{B + C} \tag{11.18}$$

Then, the estimated matched OR will be

$$\widehat{OR}_{Matched} = \frac{B/(B + C)}{1 - (B/(B + C))} = \frac{B}{C} \tag{11.19}$$

This is known as the conditional maximum likelihood estimate of the odds ratio in a (1:1) matched case–control study (Jewell, 2004). This parameter estimate can be used to give an approximation of the relative risk. For example, a hypothetical dataset is described in Table 11.11 to assess the relationship between history of smoking and myocardial infarction (MI), where the matching variables are age, sex, and physical activity.

Based on the data provided in Table 11.11,

$$\widehat{OR}_{Matched} = \frac{50}{25} = 2$$

Hence, compared to never smokers, ever smokers had a two-fold increased odds for MI. Using the program STATA (*command mcci*) we can obtain the 95% confidence interval of the $OR_{matched}$ and the McNemar test (H_0: $\pi = 0$) for this type of data (1:1) (see Table 11.12).

Table 11.11 Hypothetical number of pairs in a matched pairs (1:1) design to assess the relationship between history of smoking and myocardial infarction.

	Smoking	Controls	
		Ever	Never
Cases	Ever	200	50
	Never	25	100

Table 11.12 Example of matched analysis using McNemar's test in STATA.

```
. mcci 200 50 25 100

                    | Controls                    |
Cases               | Exposed   Unexposed  |      Total
--------------------+----------------------+------------
       Exposed |         200          50  |        250
     Unexposed |          25         100  |        125
--------------------+----------------------+------------
         Total |         225         150  |        375

McNemar's chi2(1) =        8.33    Prob > chi2 = 0.0039
Exact McNemar significance probability        = 0.0052

Proportion with factor
         Cases       .6666667
         Controls         .6      [95% Conf. Interval]
                    ---------      --------------------

         odds ratio        2        1.21409      3.3738
```

An alternative method for analyzing a matched case–control study is through a conditional logistic regression model, which can provide options for adjusting potential confounders not included in the matching criteria and the interaction assessment. This model, assuming a (1:1) design, is defined to provide the ratio of the odds of disease for two individuals from the same matched set, as follows:

$$\log \frac{p_{1k}/(1-p_{1k})}{p_{0k}/(1-p_{0k})} = \beta_E(E_{1k} - E_{ok}) + \Sigma_{j=1}^{J}\beta_j(C_{1jk} - C_{0jk}) \tag{11.20}$$

where

p_{1k} indicates the probability of disease in the kth matched set for the case given E_{1k} and C_{1k}.

p_{0k} indicates the probability of disease in the kth matched set for the control given E_{0k} and C_{0k}.

E_{1k} indicates the value of the exposure in the kth matched set for the case.

E_{0k} indicates the value of the exposure in the kth matched set for the control.

C_{1k} indicates the value of the confounding variables in the kth matched set for the case.

Table 11.13 Example of data set for conditional logistic modeling.

Pair	MI	Smoke	n
1	1	1	200
1	0	1	200
2	1	1	50
2	0	0	50
3	1	0	25
3	0	1	25
4	1	0	100
4	0	0	100

C_{0k} indicates the value of the confounding variables in the kth matched set for the control.

The process of estimating the β-parameters, often referred to as *conditional logistic regression modeling*, also yields standard errors of the estimates, which can be used to construct confidence intervals for the ORs (crude, adjusted, and for each specific stratum). To run this model, a special data set has to be prepared as shown in Table 11.13. To estimate the crude $OR_{matched}$ using the data of this table, we use the command *clogit* in STATA (see Table 11.14).

Table 11.14 Procedure to estimate the crude $OR_{matched}$ using the conditional logistic regression model.

```
. clogit mi smoke [fw=n],strata(pair) or nolog
  Conditional (fixed-effects) logistic regression
```

				Number of obs	=	750
				LR chi2(1)	=	8.49
				Prob > chi2	=	0.0036
Log likelihood = -255.68272				Pseudo R2	=	0.0163

Cases	$OR_{matched}$	OIM Std. error	z	P > |z|	95% Confidence interval	
Smoke	2.0	0.49	2.83	0.005	1.24	3.23

The results in Table 11.14 indicate that the estimated odds of MI in ever smokers is twice (95% CI: 1.24, 3.23) the odds in never smokers. These results are similar to those obtained with the *mcc* STATA command, but with a slight difference in the confidence interval.

11.15 Conclusions

In this chapter, we described the analysis of unmatched and matched case–control designs using the logistic regression model. The procedures to assess interaction terms and confounding effects are similar to those described in the previous chapter. The assessment of confounding effects is a subjective evaluation as described in the previous chapter; therefore, two researchers can arrive at different conclusions using the same set of data. Our recommendation is to use the adjusted ORs, especially if the number of confounders is small, and the results can be compared with those already published in the scientific literature. Effect modification can be evaluated using the *likelihood ratio test* for interaction terms in the model, but caution needs to be taken when the total sample size in each stratum is small. With small sample sizes, large difference in the ORs of each stratum can be observed but the *likelihood ratio test* may result in nonsignificant interaction terms in the model. Matching in case–control design presents advantages and disadvantages. Usually individual matching is useful to control the effect of known risk factors at the design level; but caution in the definition of the matching variables has to be taken to avoid over-matching. The *propensity score* has been developed to improve the matching procedure using the logistic regression model to estimate the probability of being exposed given a set of predictors. However, the traditional approach for adjustment of confounding variables, as described in this chapter, is preferable if the sample size is sufficiently large and the outcome of interest is not rare (Abadie and Imbens, 2009).

Practice Exercise

An unmatched case–control study was performed to assess the association between a diagnosis of high blood pressure (dxhigh: 1 = presence, 0 = absence) and menopausal status in 189 women. The database is as follows:

Variables	Name	Codes
Age (years)	Age	0: ≤50, 1: >50
High blood pressure	dxhigh	0: No, 1: Yes
Body mass index (kg/m^2)	bmi	0: <25, 1: ≥25
Menopause status	menop	0: premenopausal, 1: menopausal

	age	dxhigh	bmi	menop
1.	1	0	1	0
2.	1	0	1	0
3.	0	0	1	0
4.	1	0	0	1
5.	1	0	1	1
6.	0	0	0	1
7.	0	0	0	0
8.	0	0	1	0
9.	0	1	1	0
10.	1	0	1	1
11.	1	0	1	0
12.	0	1	1	0
13.	0	0	1	0
14.	0	1	1	0
15.	1	0	1	1
16.	1	0	1	1
17.	0	0	0	0
18.	0	0	0	0
19.	0	0	1	0
20.	0	0	0	0
21.	1	0	0	1
22.	1	0	1	1
23.	1	1	1	1
24.	1	1	1	1
25.	1	1	0	1
26.	1	1	0	1
27.	0	0	0	0
28.	0	0	1	0
29.	0	0	1	0
30.	1	0	1	0
31.	1	0	1	1
32.	0	0	1	0
33.	1	0	1	1
34.	0	0	1	0
35.	0	0	1	0
36.	1	0	1	1
37.	0	0	1	0
38.	0	0	1	0
39.	1	1	1	1

40.	0	0	0	0
41.	0	1	1	0
42.	0	0	0	0
43.	0	0	0	0
44.	0	0	0	0
45.	0	0	1	0
46.	0	1	0	0
47.	0	0	1	0
48.	0	0	1	0
49.	0	0	0	0
50.	0	0	1	0
51.	1	1	1	1
52.	1	1	0	1
53.	1	0	1	1
54.	0	0	0	0
55.	0	0	1	0
56.	1	0	1	0
57.	1	0	1	0
58.	1	0	1	1
59.	1	0	0	0
60.	0	0	1	0
61.	1	0	1	1
62.	1	0	1	1
63.	0	0	1	0
64.	0	0	1	0
65.	1	1	1	1
66.	0	0	1	0
67.	0	0	1	0
68.	0	0	1	0
69.	0	1	1	0
70.	0	0	0	0
71.	1	1	1	1
72.	1	1	1	1
73.	1	0	1	1
74.	1	0	1	1
75.	1	0	1	1
76.	1	1	1	1
77.	1	0	1	1
78.	0	1	1	0
79.	0	0	1	0
80.	0	0	1	0
81.	0	0	1	0
82.	0	0	0	0

83.	1	0	0	1
84.	0	0	1	0
85.	0	0	0	0
86.	1	0	0	0
87.	0	0	0	0
88.	0	0	1	0
89.	1	0	1	1
90.	1	0	1	1
91.	1	0	1	1
92.	1	0	1	1
93.	0	0	1	0
94.	1	0	1	1
95.	1	1	1	1
96.	0	1	1	0
97.	1	0	1	1
98.	0	0	0	0
99.	1	0	1	1
100.	0	0	1	1
101.	0	0	0	0
102.	0	0	1	0
103.	1	0	0	1
104.	0	0	1	0
105.	1	0	1	1
106.	0	1	1	0
107.	1	1	1	0
108.	1	1	1	1
109.	1	1	0	1
110.	0	0	1	0
111.	0	1	1	0
112.	0	0	1	0
113.	1	1	1	1
114.	0	0	0	0
115.	1	1	1	1
116.	1	1	1	0
117.	0	1	1	0
118.	1	1	1	1
119.	0	1	1	1
120.	0	0	1	0
121.	0	0	1	0
122.	0	0	1	0
123.	0	0	1	0
124.	0	0	0	0
125.	0	0	1	1

126.	1	1	1	1
127.	1	0	1	0
128.	0	0	1	0
129.	1	1	1	1
130.	1	1	1	1
131.	0	0	1	0
132.	0	0	1	0
133.	0	0	1	0
134.	0	1	1	0
135.	0	1	0	0
136.	1	1	1	0
137.	1	0	1	1
138.	0	0	1	0
139.	0	0	1	0
140.	0	0	1	0
141.	0	0	1	0
142.	0	0	1	0
143.	1	0	0	0
144.	1	0	1	1
145.	0	0	0	0
146.	1	1	1	1
147.	0	0	1	0
148.	0	1	1	0
149.	1	0	1	0
150.	0	1	1	0
151.	1	0	1	0
152.	1	0	1	1
153.	0	1	1	1
154.	1	1	1	1
155.	0	1	1	0
156.	0	0	1	0
157.	0	0	1	0
158.	1	0	0	1
159.	1	1	1	1
160.	1	1	1	1
161.	1	0	1	1
162.	1	1	0	1
163.	1	0	1	1
164.	1	0	1	1
165.	1	0	1	1
166.	0	0	1	0
167.	1	0	1	1
168.	0	0	1	0

169.	0	0	1	0
170.	0	0	0	0
171.	0	0	1	0
172.	1	1	1	1
173.	0	0	0	0
174.	0	1	1	0
175.	0	0	0	0
176.	0	0	1	0
177.	1	0	0	1
178.	1	1	1	0
179.	1	0	1	1
180.	0	0	1	1
181.	0	0	1	0
182.	1	0	1	1
183.	0	0	1	0
184.	0	0	0	0
185.	0	0	1	1
186.	0	0	1	0
187.	0	0	1	0
188.	1	1	1	0
189.	0	0	0	1

a) Estimate the magnitude of the association (odds ratio) between the diagnosis of high blood pressure and menopausal status for each age group.

b) Assess the significance of the interaction terms for menopausal status with age and body mass index in the logistic model.

c) Assuming that interaction terms were not significant, estimate the crude and adjusted odds ratios between the diagnosis of high blood pressure and menopausal status, controlling for age and body mass index.

References

Abadie, A. and Imbens, G.W. (2009) *Matching on the Estimated Propensity Score.* Working Paper Series No. 15301. Cambridge, MA: National Bureau of Economic Research.

Gordis, L. (2014) *Epidemiology*, 5th edition. Philadelphia, PA: Elsevier Saunders.

Jewell, N. (2004) *Statistics for Epidemiology*, Boca Raton, FL: Chapman & Hall/CRC.

Newman, S.C. (2001) *Biostatistical Methods in Epidemiology*. New York, NY: John Wiley & Sons, Inc.

Rothman, K.J., Greenland, S., and Lash, T.L. (2012) *Modern Epidemiology*, 3rd edition. Philadelphia, PA: Lippincott Williams & Wilkins.

Sui-Lung, S. et al. (2015) Risk factor and their interaction on chronic kidney disease: a multicenter case control study in Taiwan. *BMC Nephrol.*, **16**, 83.

Szklo, M. and Nieto, F.J. (2007) *Epidemiology Beyond the Basics*, 2nd edition. Sudbury, MA: Jones and Bartlett.

Wacholder, S. (1995) Design issues in case–control studies. *Stat. Methods. Med. Res.*, **4** (4), 293–309.

Wacholder, S., McLaughlin, J.K., Silverman, D.T., and Mandel, J.S. (1992a) Selection of controls in case–control studies: principles. *Am. J. Epidemiol.*, **135**, 1019–1028.

Wacholder, S., Silverman, D.T., McLaughlin, J.K., and Mandel, J.S. (1992b) Selection of controls in case–control studies: II. Types of controls. *Am. J. Epidemiol.*, **135**, 1029–1041.

Wacholder, S., Silverman, D.T., McLaughlin, J.K., and Mandel, J.S. (1992c) Selection of controls in case–control studies: III. Design options. *Am. J. Epidemiol.*, **135**, 1042–1050.

Woodward, M. (2014) *Epidemiology: Study Design and Data Analysis*, 3rd edition. Boca Raton, FL: Chapman & Hall.

12

Regression Models in a Cross-Sectional Study

Aim: Upon completing this chapter, the reader should be able to fit a generalized linear model for a binary and count response in a cross-sectional study design.

12.1   Introduction

A cross-sectional study design is primarily aimed at estimating the frequency of a disease or any other health-related event in a particular population or subgroups of the population at a single point in time. The study might also be useful to estimate the frequency of a particular exposure; to investigate health knowledge, attitudes, beliefs, and personal practices; or to assess health care utilization services in a population of interest (also referred to as "descriptive cross-sectional studies"). The information derived from these sort of studies is necessary for public health policy planning, allocation of health care resources, and design and implementation of public health strategies. The cross-sectional study is also used to explore the association between a particular disease or other health-related event with a variety of exposures (referred to as an "analytical cross-sectional study"). Such information can be used for the generation of hypotheses that can be tested in cohort or case–control studies.

In order to extrapolate inferences from a cross-sectional study to the target population, a random sample must be selected from the source population. There are different strategies that can be used to select this type of sample from the target population including simple random sampling, systemic sampling, stratified sampling, cluster or multistage sampling, and hybrid sampling designs (combination of these strategies). In the case of unequal probability of selection, complex sampling designs are used, particularly for sampling of households. The choice of the sampling design will depend on several factors, including the study aim, availability of a sampling frame from which participants will be selected, desired level of precision, confidence level, and budgetary constraints.

Applications of Regression Models in Epidemiology, First Edition. Erick Suárez,
Cynthia M. Pérez, Roberto Rivera, and Melissa N. Martínez.
© 2017 John Wiley & Sons, Inc. Published 2017 by John Wiley & Sons, Inc.

In some instances, random sampling designs are not used because of lack of feasibility or impracticality. In these situations, participants are selected from the target population using nonprobability sampling techniques, such as convenience sampling, judgment sampling, quota sampling, and snowball sampling techniques. Although these methods are cheaper and easier to use, the validity of inferences from nonprobability samples requires careful judgment (Heeringa et al., 2010).

Among the advantages of cross-sectional studies are their ability to estimate the prevalence of multiple attributes, lower expense and reduction in time to obtain results compared to other analytical approaches to epidemiologic studies, and their utility to investigate exposures that are fixed characteristics of individuals. Given that the study is based on prevalent cases, and not on incident cases, this design is not appropriate to investigate disease etiology nor is it suitable to investigate diseases of short duration or rare diseases or exposures. Also, since both exposure and disease are assessed simultaneously, it is difficult to establish the temporal sequence of events (Dos Santos, 1999).

12.2 Specific Objectives

- Describe the process to estimate the prevalence of selected diseases and risk factors in a cross-sectional study using a logistic regression model.
- Describe the process to estimate the magnitude of association between an exposure and disease in a cross-sectional study using the Mantel–Haenszel method.
- Describe the methods to estimate the magnitude of association between an exposure and disease using logistic and Poisson regression models.
- Compare the results obtained from the Mantel–Haenszel method and generalized linear models in a cross-sectional study.

12.3 Prevalence Estimation Using the Normal Approach

One of the important aims in a cross-sectional study is to estimate the prevalence of different attributes in the population; particularly, the prevalence of a disease or a risk factor in a community. The cross-sectional study design will depend on the manner the data are collected. The data could be collected using different random sampling designs, including simple random sampling, stratified random sampling, and cluster sampling (Levy and Lemeshow, 2009).

Simple random sampling without replacement is defined when all possible samples of size n are equally likely to be obtained from the population of size N. The sampling frame in simple random sampling usually is defined from a list individuals or enumeration units. *Stratified random sampling* occurs when each unit of the population is categorized in different strata prior to sampling; then, a simple random sampling is performed independently for each stratum. The sampling frame in this procedure is defined from a list of individuals or enumeration units in each stratum. *Cluster sampling* identifies, as a first step, a set of groups or clusters of enumeration units without making explicit the individual enumeration units. The clusters could be defined in terms of geographical areas, hospitals, schools, or clinics; these are called the primary sampling units (PSUs). One can randomly select a sample of these PSUs to obtain a list of individuals from those clusters that previously have been randomly selected. Then, for each selected cluster, a random sample of individuals could be selected using a simple random sampling.

In cross-sectional studies aimed at estimating disease prevalence, the mentioned sampling schemes are used with the limitation that the listing of individuals is not available. Therefore, a hypothetical sampling frame is defined based on U.S. Census information available from the zip codes, group of blocks of households, blocks of households, and households. As a consequence, the potential samples will not have the same probability because the PSU will have different number of individuals (i.e., number of residents in one household block will be different, or the number of persons living in one household will vary). Thus, a complex sample design is often used, combining the classical sampling designs and assigning a weight factor to each sampled individual (Heeringa et al., 2010). The weight factor may be derived as the product of the following three components: (i) probability of selection, (ii) nonresponse rate, and (iii) poststratification weight factors ("borrowing strength" from data external to the sample).

The method for drawing inference from the data generated under the sampling plan could be based on a sample design (*design-based*) or in a statistical model (*model-based*). The classical design-based procedure to estimate the prevalence of the disease using this method with 95% confidence intervals, known as the Wald interval for p, uses the *normal approach* (approximately $\hat{p} \sim N(p, (p(1-p)/n))$) as follows:

$$\hat{p} \pm 1.96^* \sqrt{\frac{\hat{p}^*(1-\hat{p})}{n}} \tag{12.1}$$

where $\hat{p} = y/n$ is the point estimate of the prevalence, y indicates the number of subjects with the attribute of interest, and n is the sample size. Another option is based on the variance stabilizing transformation for p, as follows:

$$\bar{p} = \arcsin\left(\sqrt{\hat{p}}\right) \tag{12.2}$$

The variance of $\bar{p}$ is approximately $1/(4n)$, which does not depend on p. To estimate the prevalence with 95% confidence, first a confidence interval is constructed for $\bar{p}$ $(\bar{p} \pm 1.96/\sqrt{4n})$. Then, the 95% confidence limits are converted to the original scale using the transformation $\sin(x)^2$, as follows:

$$\left(\left[\sin\left(\arcsin\sqrt{\bar{p}} - \frac{1.96}{\sqrt{4n}}\right)\right]^2, \left[\sin\left(\arcsin\sqrt{\bar{p}} + \frac{1.96}{\sqrt{4n}}\right)\right]^2\right) \tag{12.3}$$

For the model-based approach a regression model is used. For example, to construct a confidence interval for estimating the prevalence of a particular disease ($Y = 1$, given Y is a dichotomous random variable), the logistic regression model could be used without predictors as follows:

$$p_i = \frac{1}{1 + e^{-(\beta_0)}} \tag{12.4}$$

where p_i is the probability of the ith subject having the disease. The 95% confidence limits are defined as follows:

$$\left(\frac{1}{1 + e^{-(\hat{\beta}_0 - 1.96^* \mathrm{se}(\hat{\beta}_0))}}, \frac{1}{1 + e^{-(\hat{\beta}_0 + 1.96^* \mathrm{se}(\hat{\beta}_0))}}\right) \tag{12.5}$$

where $\mathrm{se}(\hat{\beta}_0)$ is the standard error of the point estimate of β_0.

For example, let us use the following data set derived from a simple random sample to estimate the prevalence of hepatitis C virus seropositivity (hcv $= 1$ denotes seropositive and hcv $= 0$ denotes seronegative) and the prevalence of cocaine use (cocaine $= 1$ denotes user, cocaine $= 0$ denotes nonuser):

Age	Cocaine	hcv
37	0	1
37	0	0
37	0	0
37	0	0
37	0	1
37	0	1
37	0	1
37	0	0
37	0	0
37	0	0
37	0	0
37	0	0
37	0	0
37	1	0
37	0	0

Age	Cocaine	hcv
37	0	1
37	0	0
37	0	0
37	0	0
37	0	0
37	0	0
37	0	0
37	0	0
37	0	0
37	0	0
38	0	0
38	1	1
38	0	0
38	0	1
38	0	0
38	0	0
38	0	0
38	0	0
38	0	0
38	0	0
38	0	0
38	0	0
38	1	1
38	0	0
38	0	0
38	0	0
38	0	0
38	1	1
38	0	0
38	0	0
38	1	0
38	0	1
38	0	0
38	0	0
38	1	1
39	0	0
39	0	0

Age	Cocaine	hcv
39	0	0
39	0	0
39	0	0
39	0	0
39	0	0
39	1	1
39	0	1
39	1	1
39	0	0
39	0	0
39	0	0
39	0	0
39	0	0
39	0	0
39	0	0
39	0	0
39	0	0
39	1	0
39	0	0
39	0	0
39	1	1

Using the Stata command *ci* with the option *Wald*, the following 95% confidence intervals are provided to estimate the prevalence for HCV and cocaine use (see Table 12.1).

Table 12.1 Example of prevalence estimation.

```
. ci proportion hcv, wald
```

Variable	Obs	Proportion	Std. error	−Binomial Wald− [95% Confidence interval]	
hcv	73	0.205	0.047	0.113	0.298

```
. ci proportion cocaine, wald
```

Variable	Obs	Proportion	Std. error	−Binomial Wald− 95% Confidence interval	
hcv	73	0.137	0.040	0.058	0.216

Based on the results of Table 12.1, the estimated prevalence of HCV seropositivity is 20.5% (95% CI: 11.3%, 29.8%) and the estimated prevalence of cocaine use is 13.7% (95% CI: 5.8%, 21.6%).

The arcsin approach can also be used with the Stata command *propci* to obtain the confidence intervals, as follows:

For HCV seropositivity:

. propcii 73 15, arcsin
Arcsin transform-based 95% CI: [0.1226, 0.3069]

For cocaine use:

. propcii 73 10, arcsin
Arcsin transform-based 95% CI: [0.0699, 0.2273]

Using the *arcsin* transformation, the estimated prevalence of HCV seropositivity is 20.5% (95% CI: 12.3%, 30.7%) and the estimated prevalence of cocaine use is 13.7% (95% CI: 7.0%, 22.7%).

Another option for prevalence estimation and obtaining confidence intervals can be performed with the logistic regression model with only the intercept (see Tables 12.2 and 12.3).

Using the results of the logistic regression model in Tables 12.2 and 12.3, the estimated prevalence of HCV seropositivity is 20.5% (95% CI: 12.8%, 31.3%) and the estimated prevalence of cocaine use is 13.7% (95% CI: 7.5%, 23.6%).

Table 12.2 Prevalence estimation of HCV with logistic regression.

```
. logistic hcv, coef

Logistic regression                    Number of obs    =       73

                                       LR chi2(0)       =     0.00

                                       Prob > chi2      =       .

Log likelihood = -37.077092            Pseudo R2        =   0.0000
```

HCV	Coef.	Std. Err.	z	P>|z|	[95% Conf. Interval]	
_cons	-1.352	0.290	-4.670	0.000	-1.920	-0.785

```
. adjust, pr ci
```

All	pr	lb	ub
	.205	.128	.313

```
Key:  pr        = Probability

      [lb , ub] = [95% Confidence Interval]
```

Table 12.3 Prevalence estimation of cocaine use with logistic regression.

```
. logistic cocaine, coef
Logistic regression                        Number of obs    =        73

                                           LR chi2(0)       =     -0.00

                                           Prob > chi2      =        .

Log likelihood = -29.160201                Pseudo R2        =    -0.0000
```

HCV	Coef.	Std. Err.	z	P>|z|	[95% Conf. Interval]	
_cons	-1.841	0.340	-5.410	0.000	-2.508	-1.173

```
. adjust, pr ci
```

All	pr	lb	ub
	.137	.075	.236

```
Key:  pr        = Probability
         [lb , ub]  = [95% Confidence Interval]
```

The confidence limits obtained from these three methods show small differences. However, if the sample size is increased, the limits will be more similar. For more information about the characteristics of the different methods to construct confidence intervals for a binomial proportion, refer to Vollset (1993).

The advantage of using the logistic regression model is that prevalence estimation can be performed for different subgroups, controlling for the effect of potential confounders. For example, the prevalence estimation of HCV seropositivity by cocaine use status, adjusted to the mean age, can be obtained with the STATA commands *logistics* and *margins* (see Table 12.4).

Using the results of the logistic regression model in Table 12.4, the estimated prevalence of HCV seropositivity among cocaine users and non-users, at mean age 38 years, is 73.4% (95% CI: 45.9, 100.0) and 11.9% (95% CI: 3.6, 20.1), respectively.

12.4 Definition of the Magnitude of the Association

In a cross-sectional study, the magnitude of the association between the exposure and disease is measured by the POR (*Prevalence Odds Ratio*). This measure is mathematically similar to the odds ratio obtained in case–control studies. The difference is in the interpretation of the *odds*. In a cross-sectional study based on a random sample, *odds* are defined based on the prevalence of an

Table 12.4 Prevalence estimation of cocaine use with logistic regression at mean age.

```
. logistic hcv i.cocaine age, coef
```

Logistic regression				Number of obs	=	73
				LR chi2(2)	=	15.10
				Prob > chi2	=	0.0005
Log likelihood = -29.528615				Pseudo R2	=	0.2036

HCV	Coef.	Std. Err.	z	P>|z|	[95% Conf. Interval]	
1.cocaine	3.0	0.85	3.55	0.000	1.354	4.689
age	-0.46	0.45	-1.03	0.303	-1.343	0.418
_cons	15.6	16.93	0.92	0.358	-17.634	48.742

```
. margins cocaine, atmeans
```

Adjusted predictions			Number of obs	=	73

```
Model VCE     : OIM
Expression    : Pr(hcv), predict()
at            : 0.cocaine    =    .8630137 (mean)
                1.cocaine    =    .1369863 (mean)
                age          =    37.9726 (mean)
```

Cocaine	Margin	Delta-method Std. Err.	z	P>|z|	[95% Conf. Interval]	
0	0.119	0.04	2.83	0.005	0.036	0.201
1	0.734	0.14	5.23	0.000	0.459	1.00

attribute in a well-defined population. For example, consider a cross-sectional study aiming to assess the magnitude of the association between age (≥ 65 years versus < 65 years) and diabetes among women, as illustrated in Table 12.5. The point estimate of the POR based on the data of Table 12.5 is

$$\widehat{POR} = \frac{\widehat{Odds}_{\geq 65}}{\widehat{Odds}_{<65}} = \frac{\hat{p}_{\geq 65}/(1-\hat{p}_{\geq 65})}{\hat{p}_{<65}/(1-\hat{p}_{<65})} = \frac{20/30}{80/270} = 2.25$$

Table 12.5 Association between age and diabetes among women.

Age	Diabetes		Total
	Present	**Absent**	
≥65 years	20	30	50
<65 years	80	270	350
Total	100	300	400

The result indicates that the prevalence *odds* of diabetes in the age group 65 years and over is 2.25 times the prevalence *odds* of diabetes in the group under 65 years.

12.5 POR Estimation

There are several methods to estimate the magnitude of the statistical association between an exposure and disease through the POR using 2×2 contingency tables. Two of these methods are Woolf's method, also referred to as the Taylor series expansion method, and the exact method.

12.5.1 Woolf's Method

To illustrate Woolf's method we will use the notation described in Table 12.6. This table is similar to the one used for a case–control study with a

Table 12.6 Notation of a 2×2 contingency table.

Exposure	Diabetes		Total
	Present	**Absent**	
Present	a	b	m_1
Absent	c	d	m_0
Total	n_1	n_0	n

a defines the number of diseased individuals among the exposed individuals.
b defines the number of nondiseased individuals among the exposed individuals.
c defines the number of diseased individuals among the unexposed individuals.
d defines the number of nondiseased individuals among the unexposed individuals.
m_1 defines the number of exposed individuals.
m_0 defines the number of unexposed individuals.
n_1 defines the number of diseased individuals.
n_0 defines the number of nondiseased individuals.
n defines the total sample size.

dichotomous exposure. In case–control studies, the marginal totals n_1 and n_0 are fixed values in the design, while in a cross-sectional study, the marginal totals (m_1, m_0, n_1, and n_0) could be random, depending on the sampling design. In a cross-sectional study, marginal totals can also be fixed when stratified sampling is used (Rosner 2010).

A point estimate of the true POR is given by ad/bc. An approximate two-sided 95% confidence interval (CI) for the POR is given by

$$\frac{ad}{bc} * e^{1.96^* \sqrt{1/a+1/b+1/c+1/d}} \tag{12.6}$$

In a cross-sectional study, to ensure an approximate normal distribution of the proportion estimate, this confidence interval should only be used if

$$m_1{}^*\hat{p}_1{}^*\hat{q}_1 > 5 \quad \text{and} \quad m_0{}^*\hat{p}_0{}^*\hat{q}_0 > 5$$

where

m_1 = the number of exposed individuals

$\hat{p}_1$ = the sample proportion with disease among exposed individuals

$\hat{q}_1 = 1 - \hat{p}_1$

m_0 = the number of unexposed individuals

$\hat{p}_0$ = the sample proportion with disease among unexposed individuals

$\hat{q}_0 = 1 - \hat{p}_0$

For example, using data from the example described in Table 12.5, the 95% CI for the population POR is given by

$$95\% \ \text{CI}: \ \frac{20 \times 270}{30 \times 80} e^{\pm 1.96 \times \sqrt{1/20+1/30+1/80+1/270}} = (1.21, \ 4.18)$$

The interval indicates that the true value of the population POR is between 1.21 and 4.18 with 95% confidence. Since the null value of the POR (H_0: POR = 1) is excluded from this interval, the data provide evidence against the null hypothesis (p-value <0.05). The syntax in Stata required to obtain this estimate is described in Table 12.7.

The data for this example meets the assumption for Woolf's method, since

$$n_1{}^*\hat{p}_1{}^*\hat{q}_1 = 50 \times 0.4 \times 0.6 = 12 > 5$$

and

$$n_2{}^*\hat{p}_2{}^*\hat{q}_2 = 350 \times 0.23 \times 0.77 = 62 > 5$$

Table 12.7 POR estimation using the Woolf method in STATA.

```
cci 20 80 30 270, w
                                                    Proportion
              | Exposed Unexposed |   Total   Exposed
--------------+-------------------+---------------------
       Cases |    20        80 |    100    0.2000
    Controls |    30       270 |    300    0.1000
--------------+-------------------+---------------------
       Total |    50       350 |    400    0.1250
              |                   |
              | Point estimate    | [95% Conf. Interval]
              |-------------------+---------------------
  Odds ratio |         2.25      | 1.212363  4.175729 (Woolf)
Attr. frac. ex. |     .5555556  | .1751647  .7605208 (Woolf)
Attr. frac. pop |     .1111111  |
              +---------------------------------------------
chi2(1) =   6.86 Pr>chi2 = 0.0088
```

12.5.2 Exact Method

To describe the exact method, we will use the notation of Table 12.8. Now assume that A defines a random variable representing the number of participants exposed among diseased individuals in the study. Then, the hypergeometric probability distribution can be used to determine the probability of $A = j$ given the four marginal totals as follows (Newman, 2001):

$$\Pr[A = j|\text{POR}] = \frac{C_j^{m_1} C_{n_1-j}^{m_0} \text{POR}^j}{\sum_u C_u^{m_1} C_{n_1-u}^{m_0} \text{POR}^u} \qquad (12.7)$$

Table 12.8 Notation of a 2×2 contingency table for the exact method.

Exposure	Disease		Total
	Present	**Absent**	
Present	j	$m_1 - j$	m_1
Absent	$n_1 - j$	$n_0 - m_1 + j$	m_0
Total	n_1	n_0	n

where $C_j^n = n!/(j!(n-j)!)$, and Σ_u indicates the sum of all values of u for which u is the maximum of 0 and (m_1-n_0), and u is the minimum of n_1 and m_1. When POR $= 1$, A has a central hypergeometric distribution, where the mass probability function is expressed as follows:

$$\Pr[A = j|\text{POR} = 1] = \frac{n_1!n_0!m_1!m_0!}{n!j!(n_1-j)!(m_1-j)!(n_0-m_1-j)!} \qquad (12.8)$$

An exact 95% confidence interval for estimating the POR is obtained by solving the two equations (Newman, 2001):

i) Determining the minimum value of the POR (POR$_L$), which fulfills the following relationship:

$$\sum_{i \geq j} \Pr[A = i|\text{POR}_L] \geq \frac{\alpha}{2}$$

ii) Determining the maximum value of the POR (POR$_U$), which fulfills the following relationship:

$$\sum_{i \leq j} \Pr[A = i|\text{POR}_U] \geq \frac{\alpha}{2}$$

The manual calculation of these limits is quite complex and time-consuming, so it is advisable to use a software package. For example, these limits can be easily determined in STATA (see Table 12.9).

Table 12.9 POR estimation using the exact method in STATA.

```
. cci 20 80 30 270, exact
                                                Proportion
                |  Exposed  Unexposed  |   Total   Exposed
  --------------+----------------------+------------------
         Cases |     20         80     |    100     0.2000
      Controls |     30        270     |    300     0.1000
  --------------+----------------------+------------------
         Total |     50        350     |    400     0.1250
                |                       |
                |   Point estimate      |  [95% Conf. Interval]
                |-----------------------+------------------
    Odds ratio |        2.25           |    1.14248  4.343039 (exact)
 Attr. frac. ex.|      .5555556         |    .1247108  .7697465 (exact)
 Attr. frac. pop|      .1111111         |
                +------------------------------------------
                        1-sided Fisher's exact P = 0.0091
                        2-sided Fisher's exact P = 0.0137]
```

The results in Table 12.9 are slightly different from those obtained in Table 12.7. However, the statistical inference is the same as above, and it is concluded that there is evidence of a statistical association between exposure and disease (p-value <0.05). Overall, the estimated prevalence odds of diabetes among the exposed group is 2.25 (95% CI: 1.14, 4.34) times the prevalence odds of diabetes among the unexposed group.

12.6 Prevalence Ratio

Another way to assess the association between an exposure and disease in a cross-sectional study is through the *prevalence ratio* (PR), a measure defined as follows (Coutinho et al., 2008):

$$PR = \frac{P_{exposed}}{P_{non-exposed}} \tag{12.9}$$

Using data from the above example, the point estimate of the PR is given by:

$$\widehat{PR} = \frac{\hat{P}_{\geq 65}}{\hat{P}_{<65}} = \frac{20/50}{80/350} = 1.75$$

This result indicates that the prevalence of diabetes among women aged 65 years and over is 1.75 times the prevalence of diabetes in women younger than 65 years. Using the normal distribution approach, the PR can be estimated using a 95% confidence interval (Agresti, 1990), as follows:

$$e^{Ln\left(\widehat{PR}\right) \pm 1.96 \times \sqrt{\frac{1}{(a+.5)} - \frac{1}{(m_1+.5)} + \frac{1}{(c+.5)} - \frac{1}{(m_0+.5)}}} \tag{12.10}$$

where a, c, m_1, and m_0 are taken from Table 12.5. $Ln\left(\widehat{PR}\right)$ is defined as follows:

$$Ln\left(\widehat{PR}\right) = Ln\left(\frac{a+.5}{m_1+.5}\right) - Ln\left(\frac{c+.5}{m_0+.5}\right)$$

Applying this formula, the 95% confidence interval (Agresti, 1990) for the PR is

$$[1.20, \ 2.60]$$

It is expected that the true value of the PR lies between 1.20 and 2.60 with 95% confidence. Therefore, there is evidence of a statistical association between age and diabetes (p-value <0.05), because the 95% confidence interval excludes the null value of the PR (H_0: PR = 1.0).

12.7 Stratified Analysis

Stratified analysis is used to evaluate the association between an exposure and disease in different subgroups of a population. In stratified analysis, subgroups or strata are defined based on the different levels of the potential confounders.

For example, if the variables age (≥ 65 years and < 65 years) and sex (male, female) are considered potential confounders in a hypothetical cross-sectional study, then four possible strata can be defined as follows:

- Stratum 1 composed of men aged 65 years or more
- Stratum 2 composed of females aged 65 years or more
- Stratum 3 composed of men under 65 years
- Stratum 4 composed of females under 65 years

Stratified analysis can be performed using different methods, such as the Mantel–Haenszel method, which is used for 2×2 contingency tables within each stratum. To illustrate this method in a cross-sectional study, a special notation is used in the 2×2 contingency table for stratum g (see Table 12.10).

The statistical analysis is performed considering the magnitude of the association in each stratum. For example, the POR in the g-th stratum is defined as follows:

$$\text{POR}_g = \frac{\text{Odds}_{\text{exposure in diseased group}}}{\text{Odds}_{\text{exposure in nondiseased group}}} = \frac{a_g/c_g}{b_g/d} = \frac{a_g{}^* d_g}{b_g{}^* c_g} \tag{12.11}$$

If the POR is different across the strata, then we conclude that there is effect modification. If there is no evidence of effect modification, a weighted POR is computed using the Mantel–Haenszel method as follows:

$$\text{POR}_{\text{MH}} = \frac{\sum_{g=1}^{G} w_g{}^* \text{POR}_g}{\sum w_g} \tag{12.12}$$

where $w_g = \frac{b_g{}^* c_g}{n_g}$

An example of the POR estimation by sex is described in Table 12.11. Based on the data from Table 12.11, the point estimate of the POR is as follows:

$$\widehat{\text{POR}}_{\text{MH}} = \frac{4.7 \times 1.66 + 1.65 \times 3.18}{4.7 + 1.65} = 2.05$$

Table 12.10 Notation of a 2×2 contingency table for stratified analysis.

Exposure	Diseased	Nondiseased	Total
Presence	a_g	b_g	$m_{1g} = a_g + b_g$
Absence	c_g	d_g	$m_{0g} = c_g + d_g$
Total	$n_{1g} = a_g + c_g$	$n_{0g} = b_g + d_g$	$n_g = a_g + b_g + c_g + d_g$

a_g is the number of diseased individuals who are exposed in stratum g.
b_g is the number of nondiseased individuals who are exposed in stratum g.
c_g is the number of diseased individuals who are non-exposed in the stratum g.
d_g is the number of nondiseased individuals who are non-exposed in the stratum g.

Table 12.11 Example of POR estimation for stratified analysis.

Sex	≥65 years		<65 years		M–H weight	$\widehat{POR}_g$
	Diabetes present	Diabetes absent	Diabetes present	Diabetes absent		
Male	13	47	20	120	$4.7 = 47 \times 20/200$	1.66
Female	7	33	10	150	$1.65 = 33 \times 10/200$	3.18
Total	20	80	30	270		

Thus, the estimated odds of having diabetes among subjects 65 years or older is 2.05 times the estimated odds of having diabetes among subjects younger than 65 years, after controlling for sex. Because both exposure and disease are assessed simultaneously, this result can be interpreted as the odds of being 65 years or older in a person with diabetes is 2.05 times the odds of being 65 years or older in a person without diabetes, after controlling for sex.

To estimate the true POR using a 95% confidence interval, the natural logarithm is used as follows (Rosner, 2010):

$$e^{\ln\left(\widehat{POR}_{MH}\right) \pm 1.96 \sqrt{Var\left(\widehat{POR}_{MH}\right)}} \qquad (12.13)$$

where

$$Var\left(\widehat{POR}_{MH}\right) = \frac{\sum_{i=1}^{k} P_i R_i}{2\left(\sum_{i=1}^{k} R_i\right)^2} + \frac{\sum_{i=1}^{k} (P_i S_i + Q_i R_i)}{2\left(\sum_{i=1}^{k} R_i\right)\left(\sum_{i=1}^{k} S_i\right)} + \frac{\sum_{i=1}^{k} Q_i S_i}{2\left(\sum_{i=1}^{k} S_i\right)^2}$$

$$P_i = \frac{a_i + d_i}{n_i}, \quad Q_i = \frac{b_i + c_i}{n_i}, \quad R_i = \frac{a_i^* d_i}{n_i}, \quad S_i = \frac{b_i^* c_i}{n_i}$$

In Stata, the 95% confidence interval can be obtained with the command *cc* (see Table 12.12).

Based on the data from Table 12.12, the excess in odds of diabetes in subjects 65 years or older compared to subjects younger than 65 years after controlling for sex is significant (95% CI: 1.1, 3.8). The estimate of the crude POR overestimates the magnitude of the association of interest. The difference in the observed point estimates of the PORs in each stratum of sex (1.66 versus 3.18) suggests the presence of effect modification in the magnitude of association of interest, which might invalidate the use of the adjusted POR. To test for homogeneity of ORs over different strata, the following statistics can be used for stratums in 2 × 2 tables, under the assumption that $H_0 : OR_1 = \cdots = OR_k$ (Rosner, 2010):

$$X_{HOM}^2 = \sum_{i=1}^{k} w_i \left(\ln\widehat{OR}_i - \overline{\ln OR}\right)^2 \qquad (12.14)$$

Table 12.12 Example of POR estimation by sex.

```
. cc diabetes age65 [fw=n], by(sex)

sex    |    OR      [95% Conf. Interval]  M-H Weight
-------------+---------------------------------------------
         1 |  1.659574    .6967565  3.831857     4.7 (exact)
         2 |  3.181818    .94684    9.987734     1.65 (exact)
-------------+---------------------------------------------
    Crude |    2.25      1.14248   4.343039          (exact)
M-H combined |  2.055118    1.10405   3.825469
-------------------------------------------------------------
```

where $\widehat{OR}_i$ indicates the point estimate of the OR in the ith stratum, and w_i indicates the weight defined for each stratum as follows:

$$w_i = \left(\frac{1}{a_i} + \frac{1}{b_i} + \frac{1}{c_i} + \frac{1}{d_i}\right)^{-1} \tag{12.15}$$

The χ^2 probability distribution is used to determine the p-value associated to X^2_{HOM}; small p-value will suggest the rejection of the ORs homogeneity. In the next section assessment of effect modification is also discussed but using the logistic regression model.

12.8 Logistic Regression Model

12.8.1 Modeling Prevalence Odds Ratio

When the aim of the cross-sectional study is to estimate the magnitude of the association between different explanatory variables and a disease (presence or absence), the following unconditional logistic regression model, described in the previous chapter, can be used (Kleinbaum, 2014):

$$\text{logit}(p_i) = \beta_0 + \sum_{j=1}^{J} \beta_j C_j \tag{12.16}$$

When we are interested in the effect of the jth predictor (X_j), assuming a dichotomous variable, the 95% confidence interval to estimate the true POR is given by the following expression:

$$POR = e^{\hat{\beta}_j \pm 1.96^* \text{se}(\hat{\beta}_j)} \tag{12.17}$$

where $\text{se}(\hat{\beta}_j)$ indicates the standard error of $\hat{\beta}_j$. Using the data from the previous example, the following data set was prepared in STATA:

```
+- - - - - - - - - - - - - - - - - - - - - - - - - +
  | diabetes    age65    sex      n |
  |- - - - - - - - - - - - - - - - - - - - - - - - -|
1. |         1        1      1     13 |
2. |         0        1      1     47 |
3. |         1        0      1     20 |
4. |         0        0      1    120 |
5. |         1        1      2      7 |
  |- - - - - - - - - - - - - - - - - - - - - - - - -|
6. |         0        1      2     33 |
7. |         1        0      2     10 |
8. |         0        0      2    150 |
+- - - - - - - - - - - - - - - - - - - - - - - - - +
```

where diabetes indicates the presence (1) or absence (0) of disease, age65 denotes the age group 1 ($\geq$65 years) and group 0 (<65 years), sex indicates whether the participant is a male (1) or female (2), and n denotes the number of participants in each of the combinations of the variables diabetes, age65, and sex.

We fitted different unconditional logistic regression models to estimate the crude, adjusted, and stratum-specific PORs and to assess the presence of interaction between age and sex (see Table 12.13).

The interpretations of the results from Table 12.13 are as follows:

Crude POR: The estimated odds of having diabetes among subjects 65 years or older is 2.3 (95% CI: 1.21, 4.18) times the estimated odds among subjects younger than 65 years. This excess in the odds of diabetes reached statistical significance (*p*-value <0.05).

Sex-Adjusted POR: The estimated odds of having diabetes among subjects 65 years or older is 2.1 (95% CI: 1.11, 3.89) times the estimated odds among

Table 12.13 POR estimation under different conditions.

		$\widehat{POR}_{\geq 65 \text{ versus } <65}$	95% CI	*p*-value
Stratum	Males	1.7	0.76, 3.60	0.20
	Females	3.2	1.13, 8.97	0.029
Crude		2.3	1.21, 4.18	0.01
Sex-adjusted*		2.1	1.11, 3.89	0.022

* No significant interaction terms were found in the model using the likelihood ratio test (*p*-value = 0.3272).

subjects younger than 65 years, adjusting for sex. This excess in the odds of diabetes reached statistical significance (*p*-value < 0.05).

Crude POR Among Males: The estimated odds of having diabetes among males 65 years or older is 1.7 (95% CI: 0.76, 3.60) times the estimated odds among males younger than 65 years. This excess in the odds of diabetes was not statistically significant (*p*-value >0.05).

Crude POR Among Females: The estimated odds of having diabetes among females 65 years or older is 3.2 (95% CI: 1.13, 8.97) times the estimated odds among females younger than 65 years. This excess in the odds of diabetes reached statistical significance (*p*-value <0.05).

Interaction Terms Assessment: Despite of the fact that the *likelihood ratio test* did not show the presence of a significant interaction between age and sex (*p*-value >0.05), the magnitude of the estimated coefficients suggest that the $\widehat{POR}_{\geq 65 \text{ versus } <65}$ among males (1.7) is quite different from the $\widehat{POR}_{\geq 65 \text{ versus } <65}$ among females (3.18); hence, sex can be considered an effect modifier.

12.8.2 Modeling Prevalence Ratio

Another procedure to estimate the magnitude of the association between different explanatory or predictor variables and a disease is the PR. For a disease that can be considered to be rare, one can estimate the PR using the following Poisson regression model:

$$\left(\frac{\mu_i}{P_i}\right) = e^{\beta_0 + \sum_{j=1}^{J} \beta_j C_j} \tag{12.18}$$

where

μ_i indicates the expected number of prevalent cases in the *i*th group.
P_i indicates the sample size in the *i*th group.
X_i indicates the predictor variables.
β_j indicates the coefficients associated with the *j*th predictor.

To estimate the PR with 95% confidence level, we use the Poisson regression model as follows:

$$PR = e^{\hat{\beta}_j \pm 1.96^* se(\hat{\beta}_j)}$$

where $\hat{\beta}_j$ indicates the point estimate of the regression coefficient associated with X_j, and $se\left(\hat{\beta}_j\right)$ indicates the standard error of $\hat{\beta}_j$. Using the previous data set, the syntax in STATA to compute the crude PR is as follows:

. glm diabetes i.age65 [fw=n], fam(poi) nolog ef							
Diabetes	Coefficient	OIM Std. error	z	P > |z|	95% Confidence interval		
1.age65	2	0.58	2.4	0.016	1.14		3.52

Interpretation: The estimated prevalence of diabetes among the age group ≥65 years is 2.0 (95% CI: 1.14, 3.52) times the estimated prevalence of diabetes among the age group <65 years.

An alternative is to use the logistic regression model with the logarithmic link function, also referred to as the log-binomial model, as follows:

. glm diabetes i.age65 [fw=n], fam(bin) nolog ef link(log)							
Diabetes	Coefficient	OIM Std. error	z	P > |z|	95% Confidence interval		
1.age65	2	0.53	2.6	0.009	1.19		3.36

Although the point estimates of the PR obtained in the log binomial and Poisson regression models are similar, there are slight differences in the standard errors of the PR. However, these differences are reduced as the sample sizes increase and with low prevalence in each exposure group.

12.9 Conclusions

The PR and POR give similar magnitudes of the association between an exposure and disease when the disease is rare. However, serious discrepancies in the measures can be observed when the prevalence in each exposure group is greater than 20%. Although the logistic regression is a commonly used technique for analyzing data from cross-sectional studies, some have argued that the prevalence ratio estimated from log-binomial, Poisson, or Cox regression models are better alternatives for the analysis of data derived from cross-sectional studies with binary outcomes (Barros and Hirakata, 2003; Petersen and Deddens, 2008). Further analysis can be performed in cross-sectional studies when correlated data are collected. Further discussion about the adjustment needed for correlated data is presented in Twisk (2013) and Snijders and Bosker (2012).

Practice Exercise

The following table summarizes the data of a cross-sectional study designed to assess the association between injection drug use (IDU) and HIV infection in males and females:

Sex	IDU	HIV positive (1)	HIV negative (0)
Male (1)	Yes (1)	137	350
	No (0)	130	543
Female (2)	Yes (1)	150	100
	No (0)	157	193

a) Estimate the crude and sex-adjusted prevalence odds ratio with a 95% confidence interval using the logistic regression model. Repeat these analyses to estimate the prevalence ratio using the Poisson regression model.
b) Estimate the prevalence odds ratio with a 95% confidence interval in males and females using the logistic regression model. Repeat these analyses to estimate the prevalence ratio using the Poisson regression model.
c) Assess the significance of the interaction term between sex and IDU in both the logistic and Poisson regression models.

References

Agresti, A. (1990) *Categorical Data Analysis*. USA: John Wiley & Sons, Ltd.

Barros, A. and Hirakata, V.N. (2003) Alternatives for logistic regression in cross-sectional studies: an empirical comparison of models that directly estimate the prevalence ratio. *BMC Med. Res. Methodol.*, **3**, 21.

Coutinho, L.M., Scazufca, M., and Menezes, P.R. (2008) Methods for estimating prevalence ratios in cross-sectional studies. *Rev. Suade Publica*, **42**, 992–998.

Dos Santos, I. (1999) *Cancer Epidemiology: Principles and Methods*. Lyon, France: World Health Organization: International Agency for Research on Cancer.

Heeringa, S.G., West, B.T., and Berglund, P.A. (2010) *Applied Survey Data Analysis*, Boca Raton, FL: Chapman & Hall/CRC.

Kleinbaum, D.G., Kupper, L.L., Nizam A., and Rosenberg E.S. (2014) *Applied regression analysis and other multivariable methods*, 5th edition. Boston, MA: Cengage Learning.

Levy, P.S. and Lemeshow, S. (2008) *Sampling of Populations: Methods and Applications*, 4th edition. John Wiley & Sons Inc. Hoboken, New Jersey.

Newman, S.C. (2001) *Biostatistical Methods in Epidemiology*, New York, NY: John Wiley & Sons, Inc.

Petersen, M.R. and Deddens, J.A. (2008) A comparison of two methods for estimating prevalence ratios. *BMC Med. Res. Methodol.*, **8**, 9.

Rosner, B. (2010) *Fundamentals of Biostatistics*, 7th edition. Boston, MA: Cengage Learning.

Snijders, T.A.B. and Bosker, R.J. (2012) *Multilevel Analysis: An Introduction to Basic and Advanced Multilevel Modeling*, 2nd edition. Thousand Oaks, CA: Sage Publications.

Twisk, J.W.R. (2013) *Applied Longitudinal Data Analysis for Epidemiology: A Practical Guide*, 2nd edition. London, UK: Cambridge University Press.

Vollset, S.E. (1993) Confidence intervals for a binomial proportion. *Stat. Med.*, **12**, 809–824.

13

Solutions to Practice Exercises

Aim: Upon completing this chapter, the reader should be able to find the codes in STATA, SAS, R, and SPSS for the practice exercises organized by chapter.

Chapter 2 Practice Exercise

In a hypothetical study, blood samples were collected in 13 children infected with malaria. The following data represent the number of parasites (*number*) found in 1 ml of blood and the age of each infant under study:

Age	Number
12	730
8	143
16	2275
8	37
11	535
10	465
12	690
13	826
15	1340
14	1580
14	1340
15	1925
15	2662

Applications of Regression Models in Epidemiology, First Edition. Erick Suárez, Cynthia M. Pérez, Roberto Rivera, and Melissa N. Martínez.
© 2017 John Wiley & Sons, Inc. Published 2017 by John Wiley & Sons, Inc.

a) Use a scatterplot to display the association between the natural logarithm of the number of parasites (response variable) and age (predictor). We recommend the use of the natural logarithm instead of the original scale because of the large variability in the data. To compute the natural logarithm of the variable number of parasites, use the *gen* and *log* commands as follows: *gen lnum = log(number).*

b) Determine and interpret the Pearson correlation between *age* and *lnum.*

c) Determine the regression line of the natural logarithm of the number of parasites as a function of age and display the results in a graph.

d) Use a graph to display the behavior of the residuals against the fitted values. How do they behave around zero? Do you see any particular pattern?

e) Based on the logarithmic model, $\hat{y}_{\ln \text{ number}} = \beta_0 + \hat{\beta}_1 \text{age}$, estimate the expected number of parasites in its original scale by age and display the results in a graph. Estimate the expected number of parasites in its original scale by age and display the results in a graph.

Question	Package	Codes
(a)	STATA	use "c2.dta", clear
		gen lnum = log (number)
		scatter lnum age
	SAS	data a;
		infile 'c2.dta';
		input age number;
		lnum=log (number);
		proc plot;
		plot lnum*age='*';
		run;
	R	data=read.table ("c2.txt", header=T)
		age=data$age
		number=data$number
		lnum=log (number)
		plot (age, lnum, pch=19)
	SPSS	**COMPUTE lnum=LN(number).**
		GRAPH/SCAT=age WITH lnum.
(b)	STATA	cor age lnum
	SAS	proc corr;
		var age lnum;
		run;
	R	cor (age, lnum)
	SPSS	**CORR age lnum.**

Question	Package	Codes
(c)	STATA	```reg lnum age```
		```predict lnesp,xb```
		```twoway (line lnesp age) (scatter lnum age)```
	SAS	```proc reg plots=none;```
		```model lnum=age;```
		```plot p.*age='*';```
		```run;```
	R	```modr=lm(lnum~age)```
		```summary(modr)```
		```plot(age,lnum, ylab="Ln(number)", pch=19)```
		```abline(modr)```
	SPSS	**REGRESSION**
		/STAT R ANOVA COEFF CI(95)
		/DEPENDENT lnum
		/METHOD=ENTER age.
		IGRAPH
		/X1=VAR(age) TYPE=SCALE
		/Y=VAR(lnum) TYPE=SCALE
		/FITLINE METHOD=REGRESSION LINEAR
		/SCATTER COINCIDENT=NONE.
(d)	STATA	```predict residual,r```
		```scatter residual lnesp, yline(0)```
	SAS	```proc reg plots=none;```
		```model lnum=age;```
		```plot r.*p.='*';```
		```run;```
	R	```residual=modr$residuals```
		```lnesp=modr$fitted.values```
		```plot(lnesp,residual,ylab="residuals",xlab="Fitted```
		```values",pch=19)```
		```abline(h=0)```
	SPSS	**REGRESSION**
		/DEPENDENT lnum
		/METHOD=ENTER age
		/SAVE PRED RESID.
		IGRAPH
		/X1=VAR(PRE_1)
		/Y=VAR(RES_1)
		/FITLINE METHOD=ORIGIN LINEAR
		/SCATTER COINCIDENT=NONE.
(e)	STATA	```gen numexp=exp(lnexp)```
		```twoway (line numexp age, sort)```
	SAS	```proc reg plots=none;```
		```model lnum=age;```

Question	Package	Codes
| | | ```
output out=fit p=yhat;
data b;
set fit;
yhatn=exp(yhat);
proc plot;
plot yhatn*age='*';
run;
``` |
| | R | ```
numexp=exp(lnexp)
dataexp=cbind(age,numexp)[order(age,numexp),]
plot(age,numexp, ylab="Fitted Values",pch=19)
lines(dataexp)
``` |
| | SPSS | ```
COMPUTE numexp=EXP(PRE_1).

GRAPH
/SCATTERPLOT(BIVAR)=age WITH numexp.
``` |

Chapter 3 Practice Exercise

The following data are concentrations of chlorophyll, phosphorus, and nitrogen taken from several lakes at different times of the day (Manly, 2001):

Lake	Chlorophyll (mg/l)	Phosphorus (mg/l)	Nitrogen (mg/l)
1	95.0	329.0	8
2	39.0	211.0	6
3	27.0	108.0	11
4	12.9	20.7	16
5	34.8	60.2	9
6	14.9	26.3	17
7	157.0	596.0	4
8	5.1	39.0	13
9	10.6	42.0	11
10	96.0	99.0	16
11	7.2	13.1	25
12	130.0	267.0	17
13	4.7	14.9	18
14	138.0	217.0	11
15	24.8	49.3	12
16	50.0	138.0	10
```

Lake	Chlorophyll (mg/l)	Phosphorus (mg/l)	Nitrogen (mg/l)
17	12.7	21.1	22
18	7.4	25.0	16
19	8.6	42.0	10
20	94.0	207.0	11
21	3.9	10.5	25
22	5.0	25.0	22
23	129.0	373.0	8
24	86.0	220.0	12
25	64.0	67.0	19

Further details of the data collection can be seen in Smith and Shapiro (1981) and Dominici et al. (1997).

a) Using matrix algebra, estimate the parameters with 95% confidence intervals of the following linear model:

$$\mu_{\text{Chlorophyll}} = \beta_0 + \beta_1 \text{ Phosphorus} + \beta_2 \text{ Nitrogen}$$

Question	Package	Codes
(a)	STATA	

```
use "c3.dta", clear
gen ones=1
mkmat ones phospho nitro, matrix(X)
mkmat chloro, matrix(chloro)
matrix INM=inv(X'*X)
matrix b=INM*X'*chloro
*Estimates of the coefficients
matrix lis b
*Calculating the MSE.
matrix MSE=(chloro'*chloro-b'*X'*chloro)/22
*Calculating the matrix of variance and covariance
matrix varb=MSE*INM
*Calculate the square root of the diagonal elements of
  varb.
mat d=cholesky(diag(vecdiag(varb)))
* Extracting the diagonal of the matrix d.
mat se=vecdiag(d)
* Show the standard error of each coefficient.
mat lis se
*95% confidence interval for phosphorus
scalar llp= b[2,1] - invttail(22, 0.025)*se[1,2]
scalar ulp= b[2,1] + invttail(22, 0.025)*se[1,2]
*95% confidence interval for nitrogen
scalar lln= b[3,1] - invttail(22, 0.025)*se[1,3]
```

Question	Package	Codes
	SAS	```scalar uln= b[3,1]+ invttail(22, 0.025)*se[1,3]```

```
scalar uln= b[3,1]+ invttail(22, 0.025)*se[1,3]
scalar list llp ulp lln uln
data a;
infile 'c3.dta';
input lake chloro phospho nitro;
proc iml;
use a;
read all var{phospho nitro} into x1;
ones=repeat(1,25,1);
x=ones||x1;
read all var{chloro} into chloro;
INM=inv(t(X)*X);
b=INM*t(X)*chloro;
print b;
MSE=(t(chloro)*chloro-t(b)*t(X)*chloro)/22;
varb=MSE*INM;
print varb;
d=sqrt(vecdiag(varb));
print d;
llp=b[2,1]-tinv(0.975,22)*d[2,1];
ulp=b[2,1]+tinv(0.975,22)*d[2,1];
print llp ulp;
lln=b[3,1]-tinv(0.975,22)*d[3,1];
uln=b[3,1]+tinv(0.975,22)*d[3,1];
print lln uln;
run;
```

R

```
data=read.table("c3.txt", header=T)
# Creating a column vector of ones, we will call "ones".
ones=rep(1,25)
# Extracting variables of the data set.
phospho=data$phospho
nitro=data$nitro
#Creating the matrix of variables.
X=cbind(ones, phospho, nitro)
#Creating the vector chloro.
chloro=data$chloro
#Calculating the inverse of the matrix
INM=solve(t(X)%*%X)
#Calculating the vector of coefficients.
b=INM%*%t(X)%*%chloro
#Show the result.
b
#Calculating the MSE.
MSE=(t(chloro)%*%chloro-t(b)%*%t(X)%*%chloro)/22
```

Question	Package	Codes

```
#Calculating the matrix of variance and covariance.
MSE=as.numeric(MSE)
varb=MSE*INM
# Show the matrix of variance and covariance.
varb
# Calculate the square root of the diagonal elements of varb.
se=sqrt(diag(varb))
# Show the standard error of each coefficient.
se
#95% confidence interval for phosphorus.
lip= b[2,1]-qt(0.975,22)*se[2]
lsp= b[2,1]+qt(0.975,22)*se[2]
# Show the limits of the interval.
lip
lsp
#95% confidence interval for nitrogen.
lin= b[3,1]-qt(0.975,22)*se[3]
lsn= b[3,1]+qt(0.975,22)*se[3]
# Show the limits of the interval.
lin
lsn
```

SPSS

```
* Opening the database in the editor.
GET
FILE='C:\Example matrixes.sav'.
* Creating a column vector of ones, call it "ones".
COMPUTE ones=1.
EXECUTE.
*Creating the matrix X of variables.
MATRIX.
GET X/VARIABLES=ONES PHOSPHO NITRO.
*Creating the vector CHLORO.
GET Y/VARIABLES=CHLORO.
* Calculate the inverse of the matrix X'X.
COMPUTE INVERSE=INV(T(X)*X).
* Calculate the coefficients vector.
COMPUTE B=INVERSE*T(X)*Y.
*Show the result.
PRINT B.
*Calculating the MSE.
COMPUTE MSE=(T(Y)*Y-T(B)*T(X)*Y)/22.
* Calculate the variance and covariance matrix
COMPUTE VARB=MSE*INVERSE.
* Show the variance and covariance matrix.
PRINT VARB.
```

Question	Package	Codes
		* Extracting the diagonal of the matrix VARB. **COMPUTE DIAGONAL=DIAG(VARB).** * Calculate the square root of the diagonal of the matrix VARB. **COMPUTE SQRTDIAG=SQRT(DIAGONAL).** * Show the standard error of each coefficient. **PRINT SQRTDIAG.** *95% confidence interval for phosphorus. **COMPUTE LLP= B(2)-(2.073873)∗SQRTDIAG(2).** **COMPUTE ULP= B(2)-(-2.073873)∗SQRTDIAG(2).** * Show the limits of the interval. **PRINT LLP.** **PRINT ULP.** **95% confidence interval for nitrogen. **COMPUTE LLN= B(3)-(2.073873)∗SQRTDIAG(3).** **COMPUTE ULN= B(3)-(-2.073873)∗SQRTDIAG(3).** * Show the limits of the interval. **PRINT LLN.** **PRINT ULN.** * End of the MATRIX syntax. **END MATRIX.**

Chapter 4 Practice Exercise

Given the information from Example 2 of this chapter to explain the level of triglycerides given waist, age and age^2 using a MLRM,

a) Make the programing in Stata, SAS, R and SPSS to evaluate the hypothesis $H_0 : \beta_2 = \beta_3 = 0_{|\text{waist}}$.

Question	Program	Codes

(a)	STATA	`use "c4.dta", clear`
		`gen age2=age^2`
		`reg trigl waist age age2`
		`test age=age2=0`

	SAS	`data a;`
		`infile 'c4.dta';`
		`age2=age*age;`
		`proc reg;`
		`model trigl=waist age age2;`
		`test age=0, age2=0;`
		`run;`

	R	`data=read.table("c4.txt", header=T)`

Question	Program	Codes
		age=data$age age2=age^2 modf=lm(trigl~waist+ age + age2, data = data) modr=lm(trigl~ waist, data = data) anova(modr, modf)
	SPSS	COMPUTE age2=age*age. REGRESSION /STATISTICS COEFF OUTS R ANOVA /DEPENDENT trigl /METHOD=TEST (waist age age2) (age age2).

Chapter 5 Practice Exercise

The body mass index (BMI) is the content of body fat in relation to height and weight of a person, which is calculated by dividing the weight of each individual in kilograms by the square of height of the individual in meters. The following table shows the BMI, age, total cholesterol, and plasma glucose of 58 adults (Pérez et al., 2008).

BMI	Age	Cholesterol	Glucose	BMI	Age	Cholesterol	Glucose
19.283	21	178	95	31.200	60	216	294
24.542	57	250	98	32.919	28	191	101
24.738	46	176	102	33.117	53	197	100
47.868	47	171	105	25.045	58	196	102
44.220	61	222	101	39.305	53	157	99
29.881	74	156	72	31.295	66	188	209
27.193	22	122	82	35.518	58	186	105
37.844	63	204	115	36.647	75	169	105
25.508	53	164	111	26.586	60	220	100
32.779	40	180	95	35.328	69	189	283
24.401	29	207	79	29.308	68	150	131
33.560	63	135	107	44.638	48	283	99
25.331	24	155	88	36.712	76	176	115
35.518	51	180	302	25.597	41	163	97
30.400	52	240	96	21.063	38	163	100
33.996	25	190	84	24.266	39	153	84
28.956	38	153	107	23.265	65	190	99
26.337	39	207	100	19.418	33	119	78

BMI	Age	Cholesterol	Glucose	BMI	Age	Cholesterol	Glucose
37.733	58	177	345	27.069	47	185	128
23.635	76	204	95	28.516	37	203	231
22.285	22	156	103	33.816	28	183	93
23.705	69	183	95	32.038	62	242	136
42.891	33	180	91	27.442	35	157	103
25.806	29	157	80	21.668	68	137	93
31.128	34	238	112	30.413	33	216	88
37.398	51	173	95	34.453	49	251	90
34.578	48	259	108	21.042	61	219	91
25.282	28	136	83	26.278	60	178	152
22.269	47	187	90	33.261	40	198	79

a) Determine the best subset of predictors that explain the variability of BMI, using the forward, backward, and stepwise methods.

Question	Program	Codes
(a)	STATA	use "c5.dta", clear
		sw reg bmi age choles glucose,pe(.05)
		sw reg bmi age choles glucose,pr(.05)
		sw reg bmi age choles glucose,pr(.1) pe(.05) forward
	SAS	data a;
		infile 'c5.dta';
		input bmi age choles glucose;
		proc reg;
		mod1: model bmi=age choles glucose/s=forward sle=0.05;
		mod2: model bmi=age choles glucose/s=backward sls=0.05;
		mod3: model bmi=age choles glucose/s=stepwise sle=0.05 sls=0.10;
		run;
	R	data=read.table("c5.txt", header=T)
		mod1=lm(bmi~choles,data=data)
		mod2=step(mod1,scope=~.+age+glucose,direction ="forward")
		mod3=lm(bmi~age+choles+glucose,data=data)
		mod2=step(mod3,scope=~.+age+glucose,direction ="backward")
		mod5=step(mod1,scope=~.+age+glucose,direction ="both")

Question	Program	Codes
	SPSS	REGRESSION /STATISTICS COEFF OUTS R ANOVA /DEPENDENT bmi /METHOD=FORWARD age choles glucose. REGRESSION /STATISTICS COEFF OUTS R ANOVA /DEPENDENT bmi /METHOD=BACKWARD age choles glucose. REGRESSION /STATISTICS COEFF OUTS R ANOVA /DEPENDENT bmi /METHOD=STEPWISE age choles glucose.

Chapter 6 Practice Exercise

Using the previous database, determine the correlation between *triglycerides* and *cholesterol* levels when

a) controlling for *hemoglogin* levels,
b) controlling for *hemoglobin* and *glucose* levels
c) only *cholesterol* is controlled for *hemoglobin* levels and *weight*.

Question	Program	Codes
(a)	STATA	use "c6.dta", clear quietly: reg trigl hemog predict r1, r quietly: reg choles hemog predict r2, r corr r1 r2 *option with pcorrmat pcorrmat trigl choles, part(hemog)
	SAS	data a; infile 'c6.dta'; input weight choles hemog trigl gluco; proc corr nosimple; var trigl choles; partial hemog; run;
	R	data=read.table("c6.txt", header=T) mod1=lm(trigl~hemog,data=data)

Question	Program	Codes

		```resid1=mod1$residuals```
		```mod1=lm(choles~hemog,data=data)```
		```resid2=mod1$residuals```
		```cor(resid1,resid2)```

	SPSS	```REGRESSION```
		```/DEPENDENT trigl```
		```/METHOD=ENTER hemog```
		```/SAVE resid1.```

		```REGRESSION```
		```/DEPENDENT choles```
		```/METHOD=ENTER hemog```
		```/SAVE resid2.```

		```CORRELATIONS```
		```/VARIABLES=RES_1 RES_2```
		```/PRINT=TWOTAIL NOSIG```
		```/MISSING=PAIRWISE.```

(b)	STATA	```quietly: reg trigl hemog gluco```
		```predict r3, r```
		```quietly: reg choles hemog gluco```
		```predict r4, r```
		```corr r3 r4```
		```*option with pcorrmat```
		```pcorrmat trigl choles, part(hemog gluco)```

	SAS	```proc corr nosimple;```
		```var trigl choles;```
		```partial hemog gluco;```
		```run;```

	R	```mod1=lm(trigl~hemog+gluco,data=data)```
		```resid3=mod1$residuals```
		```mod1=lm(choles~hemog+gluco,data=data)```
		```resid4=mod1$residuals```
		```cor(resid3,resid4)```

	SPSS	```REGRESSION```
		```/DEPENDENT trigl```
		```/METHOD=ENTER hemog gluco```
		```/SAVE resid3.```

		```REGRESSION```
		```/DEPENDENT choles```
		```/METHOD=ENTER hemog gluco```
		```/SAVE resid4.```

		```CORRELATIONS```
		```/VARIABLES=res_3 res_4```
		```/PRINT=TWOTAIL NOSIG```
		```/MISSING=PAIRWISE.```

Question	Program	Codes
(c)	STATA	**quietly: reg choles hemog weight** **predict r5, r** **corr trigl r5**

	SAS	`proc reg noprint plots=none;`
		`model choles=hemog weight;`
		`output out=stats r=residual;`
		`proc corr;`
		`var trigl residual;`
		`run;`

	R	`mod1=lm(choles~hemog+weight,data=data)`
		`resid5=mod1$residuals`
		`trigl=data$trigl`
		`cor(trigl, resid5)`

	SPSS	`REGRESSION`
		`/DEPENDENT choles`
		`/METHOD=ENTER hemog weight`
		`/SAVE resid5.`
		
		`CORRELATIONS`
		`/VARIABLES=trigl RES_5`
		`/PRINT=TWOTAIL NOSIG.`

Chapter 7 Practice Exercise

Some studies have shown a positive relationship between the amount of ozone in the air and increased mortality from circulatory and respiratory diseases. Using the following data, fit a regression model for predicting ozone levels as a function of the amount of solar radiation, temperature, and wind speed.

Ozone	Radiation	Temperature	Wind speed	Ozone	Radiation	Temperature	Wind speed
2.76	230	75	10.9	4.31	294	86	8.6
2.76	259	76	15.5	4.86	223	79	5.7
4.00	253	83	7.4	3.33	279	76	7.4
4.79	207	90	8.0	2.84	14	71	9.2
3.11	322	68	11.5	4.90	225	94	2.3
4.00	175	83	4.6	3.68	275	86	7.4
2.52	7	74	6.9	3.39	83	81	6.9
3.94	285	84	6.3	3.56	212	79	9.7
3.42	314	83	10.9	2.52	77	82	7.4
4.27	197	92	5.1	2.35	27	76	10.3

Ozone	Radiation	Temperature	Wind speed	Ozone	Radiation	Temperature	Wind speed
3.39	323	87	11.5	3.33	284	72	20.7
3.11	193	70	6.9	2.62	131	76	8.0
2.35	238	64	12.6	4.25	276	88	5.1
4.50	189	93	4.6	3.45	190	67	7.4
3.61	95	87	7.4	4.14	291	90	13.8

a) Graph the jackknife residuals distribution using a normal quantile plot.
b) Graph the leverage values against the observation's identification number (id), indicating the suggested limit for influential values.
c) Graph the statistic DFFITS, indicating the suggested limit for influential values.

Question	Program	Codes
(a)	STATA	use "c7.dta", clear quietly: reg ozone radiation temp wind predict rjk, rstudent qnorm rjk, title(Normality Plot)

	SAS	data a;
		infile 'c7.dta';
		input ozone radiation temp wind;
		id=_n_;
		proc reg noprint;
		model ozone=radiation temp wind;
		plot rstudent.*nqq.;
		run;

	R	data=read.table("c7.txt", header=T) mod=lm(ozone~radiation + temp + wind,data=data) rjk=rstudent(mod) qqnorm(rjk, main="Normality Plot") qqline(rjk)
	SPSS	REGRESSION /STATISTICS COEFF OUTS R ANOVA /DEPENDENT ozone /METHOD=ENTER radiation temp wind /SAVE SDRESID. EXAMINE VARIABLES=SDR_1 /PLOT NPPLOT /STATISTICS NONE /CINTERVAL 95 /NOTOTAL.

Question	Program	Codes

(b)	STATA	```predict l, lev```
		```gen id=_n```
		```twoway(scatter l id), yline(0.267)```

	SAS	```proc reg noprint;```
		```model ozone=radiation temp wind;```
		```output out=stats h=leverage;```
		```data b;```
		```set stats;```
		```proc plot;```
		```plot leverage*id='*'/vref=0.267;```
		```run;```

	R	```lev=hatvalues(mod)```
		```plot(lev)```
		```abline(h=0.267)```

	SPSS	```REGRESSION```
		```/STATISTICS COEFF OUTS R ANOVA```
		```/DEPENDENT ozone```
		```/METHOD=ENTER radiation temp wind```
		```/SAVE LEVER.```
		```COMPUTE id=$CASENUM.```
		```FORMAT id (F8.0).```
		```EXECUTE.```
		
		```GRAPH```
		```/SCATTERPLOT(BIVAR)=id WITH LEV_1.```

(c)	STATA	```predict ozonefit,dfits``` ```scatter ozonefit id, mlabel(id) yline(.52)```

	SAS	```proc reg noprint;```
		```model ozone=radiation tempe wind;```
		```output out=stats dffits=dffits;```
		```data b;```
		```set stats;```
		```proc plot;```
		```plot dffits*id='*'/vref=0.52;```
		```run;```

	R	```dfit=dffits(mod)``` ```plot(dfit)```

	SPSS	```REGRESSION```
		```/STATISTICS COEFF OUTS R ANOVA```
		```/DEPENDENT ozone```
		```/METHOD=ENTER radiation temp wind```
		```/SAVE DFFIT.```
		
		```GRAPH```
		```/SCATTERPLOT(BIVAR)=id WITH DFF_1.```

Chapter 8 Practice Exercise

Suppose we are interested in predicting the weight in premature children by gestational age. The following table presents the average weight (in grams) and the gestational age (in weeks) of 100 children with low birth weight.

Weight	Gestation	r
670.0	23	2
795.0	24	2
715.7	25	7
907.0	26	5
981.4	27	14
1075.5	28	11
1141.5	29	20
1151.5	30	13
1257.3	31	11
1266.0	32	5
1368.8	33	8
1440.0	34	1
1490.0	35	1

a) Fit a regression model to explain the weight by gestational age without using the number of births as a weighting factor.
b) Using the previous model, display the residuals against the fitted values.
c) Fit a regression model to explain the weight as a function of gestational age using the number of births as a weighting factor.
d) Using the previous model, display the residuals against the fitted values.

Question	Program	Codes
(a)	STATA	`use "c8.dta", clear` `reg weight gesta`

	SAS	`data a;`
		`infile 'c8.dta';`
		`input weight gesta r;`
		`proc reg;`
		`model weight=gesta;`
		`run;`

	R	`data=read.table("c8.txt", header=T)`
		`mod=lm(weight~gesta,data=datap)`
		`summary(mod1)`

Question	Program	Codes
| | SPSS | ```
REGRESSION
/STATISTICS COEFF OUTS R ANOVA
/DEPENDENT weight
/METHOD=ENTER gesta.
``` |
| (b) | STATA | ```
predict weiexp
predict res,r
twoway(scatter res weiexp), yline(0)
``` |
| | SAS | ```
proc reg noprint plots(only label)=
    (ResidualByPredicted);
model weight=gesta;
run;
``` |
| | R | ```
res=mod$residuals
weiexp=mod$fitted.values
plot(weiexp, res)
abline(h=0)
``` |
| | SPSS | ```
REGRESSION
/STATISTICS COEFF OUTS R ANOVA
/DEPENDENT weight
/METHOD=ENTER gesta
/SAVE PRED RESID.
GRAPH
/SCATTERPLOT(BIVAR)=PRE_1 WITH RES_1.
``` |
| (c) | STATA | ```
gen w=sqrt(r)
gen gesta2=gesta*w
gen weight2=weight*w
reg weight2 gesta2 w, noconst
``` |
| | SAS | ```
data b;
set a;
w=sqrt(r);
gesta2=gesta*w;
weight2=weight*w;
proc reg plots=none;
model weight2=gesta2 w/noint;
run;
``` |
| | R | ```
weight=data$weight
gesta=data$gesta
r=data$r
w=sqrt(r)
gesta2=gesta*w
weight2=weight*w
mod2=lm(weight2~gesta2+w-1)
summary(mod2)
``` |
| | SPSS | ```
COMPUTE w=SQRT(r).
COMPUTE gesta2=gesta*w.
``` |
```

Question	Program	Codes
		EXECUTE.
		COMPUTE weight2=weight*w.
		EXECUTE.
		REGRESSION
		/ORIGIN
		/STATISTICS COEFF OUTS R ANOVA
		/DEPENDENT weight2
		/METHOD=ENTER gesta2 w.
(d)	STATA	predict weiexp2
		predict res2,r
		twoway (scatter res2 weiexp2), yline(0)
	SAS	proc reg noprint plots(only label)=
		(ResidualByPredicted);
		model weight2=gesta2 w/noint;
		run;
	R	res2=mod2$residuals
		weiexp2=mod2$fitted.values
		plot(weiexp2,res2)
		abline(h=0)
	SPSS	REGRESSION
		/ORIGIN
		/STATISTICS COEFF OUTS R ANOVA
		/DEPENDENT weight2
		/METHOD=ENTER gesta2 w
		/SAVE PRED RESID.
		GRAPH
		/SCATTERPLOT(BIVAR)=PRE_2 WITH RES_2.

Chapter 10 Practice Exercise

The following table summarizes the data of a cohort study designed to test the hypothesis that obesity increases the risk of cardiovascular disease (CVD):

Age in years	Obesity	CVD	Person-years
60–64	Obese	10	245
	Not obese	12	640
65–69	Obese	34	365
	Not obese	45	520
70–74	Obese	40	250
	Not obese	44	490

a) Evaluate the significance of the interaction between age and obesity using a Poisson regression model.
b) Estimate the relative risk of CVD according to obesity using a 95% confidence interval.
c) Estimate the relative risk of CVD according to obesity for each age group using a 95% confidence interval.
d) Estimate the relative risk of CVD according to obesity status adjusting for age group using a 95% confidence interval.

Question	Program	Codes

(a)	STATA	```use "c10.dta", clear```
		```quietly xi: glm cvd i.obese*i.age, fam(poi) lnoff(pys)```
		```estimate store model1```
		```quietly xi: glm cvd i.obese i.age, fam(poi) lnoff(pys)```
		```lrtest model1 .```

	SAS	```data a;```
		```infile 'c10.dta';```
		```input age obese cvd pys;```
		```proc genmod;```
		```class age (ref='1') obese (ref='0')/param=effect;```
		```model cvd=obese|age/link=log dist=poi offset=lpy;```
		```contrast 'interaction' obese*age 1 1, obese*age 0 1;```
		```run;```

	R	```data=read.table("c10.txt", header=T)```
		```age=c(1,1,2,2,3,3)```
		```age=factor(age)```
		```obese=c(1,0,1,0,1,0)```
		```cvd=c(10,12,34,45,40,44)```
		```pys=c(245,640,365,520,250,490)```
		```data_b=data.frame(age=age,obese=obese,cvd=cvd,```
		``` pys=pys)```
		```mod1=glm(cvd~obese+age,family=poisson,offset=log```
		``` (pys),data=data_b)```
		```mod2=glm(cvd~obese*age,family=poisson,offset=log```
		``` (pys),data=data_b)```
		```anova(mod1,mod2,test="LRT")```

	SPSS	```COMPUTE lpy=ln(pys).```
		
		```GENLIN cvd BY age obese (ORDER=ASCENDING)```
		```/MODEL age obese age*obese INTERCEPT=YES OFFSET=lpy```
		```DISTRIBUTION=POISSON LINK=LOG```
		```/PRINT MODELINFO SUMMARY.```

(b)	STATA	```xi: glm cvd i.obese, fam(poi) lnoff(pys) ef```
	SAS	```proc genmod;``` ```class obese (ref='0');```

Question	Program	Codes
		```model cvd=obese/link=log dist=poi offset=lpy;```
		```estimate `IRR' obese 1 -1;```
		```run;```
	R	```mod=glm(cvd~obese,family=poisson,offset=log(pys),```
		``` data=data_b)```
		```exp(confint(mod))```
	SPSS	```GENLIN cvd BY obese (ORDER=DESCENDING)```
		```/MODEL obese OFFSET=lpy```
		```DISTRIBUTION=POISSON LINK=LOG```
		```/PRINT MODELINFO SOLUTION(EXPONENTIATED).```
(c)	STATA	```xi: glm cvd i.obese if age==1, fam(poi) lnoff(pys) ef```
		```xi: glm cvd i.obese if age==2, fam(poi) lnoff(pys) ef```
		```xi: glm cvd i.obese if age==3, fam(poi) lnoff(pys) ef```
	SAS	```proc sort; by age;```
		```proc genmod;```
		```class obese (ref='0');```
		```model cvd=obese/link=log dist=poi offset=lpy;```
		```by age;```
		```estimate 'IRR' obese 1 -1;```
		```run;```
	R	```mods=glm(cvd~obese,family=poisson,offset=log(pys),```
		``` data=data_b[age==1,])```
		```exp(confint(mods))```
		```mods=glm(cvd~obese,family=poisson,offset=log(pys),```
		``` data=data_b[age==2,])```
		```exp(confint(mods))```
		```mods=glm(cvd~obese,family=poisson,offset=log(pys),```
		``` data=data_b[age==3,])```
		```exp(confint(mods))```
	SPSS	```TEMPORARY.```
		```SELECT IF (age=1).```
		```GENLIN cvd BY obese (ORDER=DESCENDING)```
		```/MODEL obese OFFSET=lpy```
		```DISTRIBUTION=POISSON LINK=LOG```
		```/PRINT MODELINFO SOLUTION(EXPONENTIATED).```
		```TEMPORARY.```
		```SELECT IF (age=2).```
		```GENLIN cvd BY obese (ORDER=DESCENDING)```
		```/MODEL obese OFFSET=lpy```
		```DISTRIBUTION=POISSON LINK=LOG```
		```/PRINT MODELINFO SOLUTION(EXPONENTIATED).```
		```TEMPORARY.```
		```SELECT IF (age=3).```
		```GENLIN cvd BY obese (ORDER=DESCENDING)```

Question	Program	Codes
		`/MODEL obese OFFSET=lpy`
		`DISTRIBUTION=POISSON LINK=LOG`
		`/PRINT MODELINFO SOLUTION(EXPONENTIATED).`
(d)	STATA	`xi: glm cvd i.obese i.age, fam(poi) lnoff(pys) ef`
	SAS	`proc genmod;`
		`class age (ref='1') obese (ref='0');`
		`model cvd=obese age/link=log dist=poi offset=lpy;`
		`estimate 'IRR' obese 1 -1;`
		`run;`
	R	`modadj=glm(cvd~obese+age,family=poisson,offset=log`
		`    (pys),data=data_b)`
		`exp(confint(modadj))`
	SPSS	`GENLIN cvd BY obese age (ORDER=ASCENDING)`
		`/MODEL obese age OFFSET=lpy`
		`DISTRIBUTION=POISSON LINK=LOG`
		`/PRINT MODELINFO SOLUTION(EXPONENTIATED).`

Chapter 11 Practice Exercise

An unmatched case–control study was performed to assess the association between a diagnosis of high blood pressure (dxhigh: 1=presence, 0=absence) and menopausal status in 189 women. The database is the following:

Variables	Name	Codes
Age (years)	Age	0: ≤50, 1: >50
High blood pressure	dxhigh	0: No, 1: Yes
Body mass index	bmi	0: <25, 1: ≥25
Menopause status	menop	0: premenopausal, 1: menopausal

	age	dxhigh	bmi	menop
1.	1	0	1	0
2.	1	0	1	0
3.	0	0	1	0
4.	1	0	0	1
5.	1	0	1	1
6.	0	0	0	1

7.	0	0	0	0
8.	0	0	1	0
9.	0	1	1	0
10.	1	0	1	1
11.	1	0	1	0
12.	0	1	1	0
13.	0	0	1	0
14.	0	1	1	0
15.	1	0	1	1
16.	1	0	1	1
17.	0	0	0	0
18.	0	0	0	0
19.	0	0	1	0
20.	0	0	0	0
21.	1	0	0	1
22.	1	0	1	1
23.	1	1	1	1
24.	1	1	1	1
25.	1	1	0	1
26.	1	1	0	1
27.	0	0	0	0
28.	0	0	1	0
29.	0	0	1	0
30.	1	0	1	0
31.	1	0	1	1
32.	0	0	1	0
33.	1	0	1	1
34.	0	0	1	0
35.	0	0	1	0
36.	1	0	1	1
37.	0	0	1	0
38.	0	0	1	0
39.	1	1	1	1
40.	0	0	0	0
41.	0	1	1	0
42.	0	0	0	0
43.	0	0	0	0
44.	0	0	0	0
45.	0	0	1	0
46.	0	1	0	0
47.	0	0	1	0
48.	0	0	1	0
49.	0	0	0	0

50.	0	0	1	0
51.	1	1	1	1
52.	1	1	0	1
53.	1	0	1	1
54.	0	0	0	0
55.	0	0	1	0
56.	1	0	1	0
57.	1	0	1	0
58.	1	0	1	1
59.	1	0	0	0
60.	0	0	1	0
61.	1	0	1	1
62.	1	0	1	1
63.	0	0	1	0
64.	0	0	1	0
65.	1	1	1	1
66.	0	0	1	0
67.	0	0	1	0
68.	0	0	1	0
69.	0	1	1	0
70.	0	0	0	0
71.	1	1	1	1
72.	1	1	1	1
73.	1	0	1	1
74.	1	0	1	1
75.	1	0	1	1
76.	1	1	1	1
77.	1	0	1	1
78.	0	1	1	0
79.	0	0	1	0
80.	0	0	1	0
81.	0	0	1	0
82.	0	0	0	0
83.	1	0	0	1
84.	0	0	1	0
85.	0	0	0	0
86.	1	0	0	0
87.	0	0	0	0
88.	0	0	1	0
89.	1	0	1	1
90.	1	0	1	1
91.	1	0	1	1
92.	1	0	1	1

93.	0	0	1	0
94.	1	0	1	1
95.	1	1	1	1
96.	0	1	1	0
97.	1	0	1	1
98.	0	0	0	0
99.	1	0	1	1
100.	0	0	1	1
101.	0	0	0	0
102.	0	0	1	0
103.	1	0	0	1
104.	0	0	1	0
105.	1	0	1	1
106.	0	1	1	0
107.	1	1	1	0
108.	1	1	1	1
109.	1	1	0	1
110.	0	0	1	0
111.	0	1	1	0
112.	0	0	1	0
113.	1	1	1	1
114.	0	0	0	0
115.	1	1	1	1
116.	1	1	1	0
117.	0	1	1	0
118.	1	1	1	1
119.	0	1	1	1
120.	0	0	1	0
121.	0	0	1	0
122.	0	0	1	0
123.	0	0	1	0
124.	0	0	0	0
125.	0	0	1	1
126.	1	1	1	1
127.	1	0	1	0
128.	0	0	1	0
129.	1	1	1	1
130.	1	1	1	1
131.	0	0	1	0
132.	0	0	1	0
133.	0	0	1	0
134.	0	1	1	0
135.	0	1	0	0

136.	1	1	1	0
137.	1	0	1	1
138.	0	0	1	0
139.	0	0	1	0
140.	0	0	1	0
141.	0	0	1	0
142.	0	0	1	0
143.	1	0	0	0
144.	1	0	1	1
145.	0	0	0	0
146.	1	1	1	1
147.	0	0	1	0
148.	0	1	1	0
149.	1	0	1	0
150.	0	1	1	0
151.	1	0	1	0
152.	1	0	1	1
153.	0	1	1	1
154.	1	1	1	1
155.	0	1	1	0
156.	0	0	1	0
157.	0	0	1	0
158.	1	0	0	1
159.	1	1	1	1
160.	1	1	1	1
161.	1	0	1	1
162.	1	1	0	1
163.	1	0	1	1
164.	1	0	1	1
165.	1	0	1	1
166.	0	0	1	0
167.	1	0	1	1
168.	0	0	1	0
169.	0	0	1	0
170.	0	0	0	0
171.	0	0	1	0
172.	1	1	1	1
173.	0	0	0	0
174.	0	1	1	0
175.	0	0	0	0
176.	0	0	1	0
177.	1	0	0	1
178.	1	1	1	0

179.	1	0	1	1
180.	0	0	1	1
181.	0	0	1	0
182.	1	0	1	1
183.	0	0	1	0
184.	0	0	0	0
185.	0	0	1	1
186.	0	0	1	0
187.	0	0	1	0
188.	1	1	1	0
189.	0	0	0	1

a) Estimate the magnitude of the association (odds ratio) between the diagnosis of high blood pressure and menopausal status for each age group.
b) Assess the significance of the interaction terms for menopausal status with age and body mass index in the logistic model.
c) Assuming that interaction terms were not significant, estimate the crude and adjusted odds ratios between the diagnosis of high blood pressure and menopausal status, controlling for age, and body mass index.

Question	Program	Codes
(a)	STATA	use "c11.dta", clear xi: glm dxhigh i.menop if age==0, fam(bin) ef xi: glm dxhigh i.menop if age==1, fam(bin) ef

	SAS	data a;
		infile 'c11.dta';
		input age dxhigh bmi menop;
		proc sort; by age;
		proc logistic descending;
		class menop (ref='0');
		model dxhigh=menop;
		by age;
		run;

	R	data=read.table("c11.txt", header=T) age=data$age age=factor(age) bmi=data$bmi bmi=factor(bmi) menop=data$menop menop=factor(menop) mods=glm(dxhigh~menop,family=binomial,data=data [age==0,]) exp(confint(mods))

Question	Program	Codes

		`mods=glm(dxhigh~menop,family=binomial,data=data`
		`  [age==1,])`
		`exp(confint(mods))`

	SPSS	`LOGISTIC REGRESSION VARIABLES = dxhigh WITH menop`
		`/PRINT = ci(95)`
		`/SELECT=age=0.`
		`LOGISTIC REGRESSION VARIABLES = dxhigh WITH menop`
		`/PRINT = ci(95)`
		`/SELECT=age=1.`

(b)	STATA	`quietly xi: glm dxhigh i.meno*i.age i.meno*i.bmi, fam`
		`  (bin)`
		`estimate store model1`
		`quietly xi: glm dxhigh i.meno i.age i.bmi, fam(bin)`
		`lrtest model1 .`

	SAS	`proc logistic descending;`
		`class menop (ref='0') age (ref='0') bmi(ref='0');`
		`model dxhigh=menop age bmi menop*age menop*bmi;`
		`contrast 'interactions' menop*age 1, menop*bmi 1;`
		`run;`

	R	`mod=glm(dxhigh~menop+age+bmi,family=binomial,`
		`  data=data)`
		`mod_1=glm(dxhigh~menop*age + menop*bmi,`
		`  family=binomial,data=data)`
		`anova(mod,mod_1,test="LRT")`

	SPSS	`LOGISTIC REGRESSION VAR dxhigh WITH menop age bmi`
		`/CATEGORICAL menop age bmi`
		`/METHOD=ENTER menop age bmi menop*age menop*bmi`
		`/PRINT SUMMARY .`

(c)	STATA	`xi: glm dxhigh i.meno, fam(bin) ef` `xi: glm dxhigh i.meno i.age i.bmi, fam(bin) ef`

	SAS	`proc logistic descending;`
		`class menop (ref='0');`
		`model dxhigh=menop;`
		`proc logistic descending;`
		`class menop (ref='0') age (ref='0') bmi (ref='0');`
		`model dxhigh=menop age bmi;`
		`run;`

	R	`mod_c=glm(dxhigh~menop,family=binomial,data=data)`
		`exp((mod_c$coefficients[2]))`
		`exp(confint(mod_c))`
		`mod_a=glm(dxhigh~menop+age+bmi,family=binomial,`
		`  data=data)`
		`exp((mod_a$coefficients[2]))`
		`exp(confint(mod_a))`

Question	Program	Codes
	SPSS	LOGISTIC REGRESSION VAR = dxhigh WITH menop /PRINT = ci(95). LOGISTIC REGRESSION VAR = dxhigh WITH menop age bmi /PRINT = ci(95).

Chapter 12 Practice Exercise

The following table summarizes the data of a cross-sectional study designed to assess the association between HIV infection and injection drug use (IDU) in males and females:

Sex	IDU	HIV positive	HIV negative
Male	Yes	137	350
	No	130	543
Female	Yes	150	100
	No	157	193

a) Estimate the crude and sex-adjusted prevalence odds ratio with a 95% confidence interval using the logistic regression model. Repeat these analyses to estimate the prevalence ratio using the Poisson regression model.
b) Estimate the prevalence odds ratio with a 95% confidence interval in males and females using the logistic regression model. Repeat these analyses to estimate the prevalence ratio using the Poisson regression model.
c) Assess the significance of the interaction term between sex and IDU in both the logistic and Poisson regression models.

Question	Program	Codes
(a)	STATA	use "c12.dta", clear gen total=hivpos+hivneg *Logistic regression xi: glm hivpos i.idu, fam(bin total) ef xi: glm hivpos i.idu i.sex, fam(bin total) ef *Poisson regression model xi: glm hivpos i.idu, fam(poi) lnoff(total) ef xi: glm hivpos i.idu i.sex, fam(poi) lnoff(total) ef
	SAS	data j; infile 'c12.dta';

Question	Program	Codes

```
                      input sex idu hivpos hivneg;
                      total=hivpos+hivneg;
                      proc logistic descending;
                      class idu (ref='0');
                      model hivpos/total=idu;
                      proc logistic descending;
                      class idu (ref='0') sex (ref='1');
                      model hivpos/total=idu sex;
                      proc genmod;
                      class idu (ref='0');
                      model hivpos/total=idu/link=log dist=poi;
                      estimate 'Unadjusted PR' idu 1 -1;
                      proc genmod;
                      class idu (ref='0') sex (ref='1');
                      model hivpos/total=idu sex/link=log dist=poi;
                      estimate 'Adjusted PR' idu 1 -1;
                      run;
```

	R	

```
                      data=read.table("c12.txt", header=T)
                      hivpos=data$hivpos
                      hivneg=data$hivneg
                      idu=data$idu
                      sex=data$sex
                      modbi=glm(cbind(hivpos,hivneg)~idu,family=binomial,
                        data=data)
                      exp((modbi$coefficients[2]))
                      exp(confint(modbi))
                      modbc=glm(cbind(hivpos,hivneg)~idu + sex,
                        family=binomial,data=data)
                      exp((modbc$coefficients[2]))
                      exp(confint(modbc))
                      total= hivpos+hivneg
                      modpi=glm(hivpos~idu,family=poisson, offset=log
                        (total), data=data)
                      exp((modpi$coefficients[2]))
                      exp(confint(modpi))
                      modpc=glm(hivpos~idu+sex,family=poisson, offset=log
                        (total), data=data)
                      exp((modpc$coefficients[2]))
                      exp(confint(modpc))
```

	SPSS	*Logistic regression

```
                      COMPUTE total=hivpos+hivneg.

                      GENLIN hivpos OF total BY idu (ORDER=DESCENDING)
                      /MODEL idu
                      DISTRIBUTION=binomial LINK=LOGIT
```

Question	Program	Codes

```
/PRINT MODELINFO SOLUTION (EXPONENTIATED).

GENLIN hivpos OF total BY idu sex (ORDER=DESCENDING)
/MODEL idu sex
DISTRIBUTION=binomial LINK=LOGIT
/PRINT MODELINFO SOLUTION (EXPONENTIATED).
```

** Poisson model

```
COMPUTE ltotal=ln(total).

GENLIN hivpos BY idu (ORDER=DESCENDING)
/MODEL idu OFFSET=ltotal
DISTRIBUTION=POISSON LINK=LOG
/PRINT MODELINFO SOLUTION (EXPONENTIATED).
GENLIN hivpos BY idu sex (ORDER=DESCENDING)
/MODEL idu sex OFFSET=ltotal
DISTRIBUTION=POISSON LINK=LOG
/PRINT MODELINFO SOLUTION (EXPONENTIATED).
```

Question	Program	Codes

(b)	STATA	```xi: glm hivpos i.idu if sex==1,fam(bin total) ef```
		```xi: glm hivpos i.idu if sex==2,fam(bin total) ef```
		```xi: glm hivpos i.idu if sex==1,fam(poi) lnoff(total) ef```
		```xi: glm hivpos i.idu if sex==2,fam(poi) lnoff(total) ef```

	SAS	```proc sort; by sex;```
		```proc logistic descending;```
		```class idu (ref='0');```
		```model hivpos/total=idu;```
		```by sex;```
		```proc genmod;```
		```class idu (ref='0');```
		```model hivpos/total=idu/link=log dist=poi;```
		```by sex;```
		```estimate 'Unadjusted PR' idu 1 -1;```
		```run;```

	R	```modbs1=glm(cbind(hivpos,hivneg) ~idu,```
		``` family=binomial,```
		```data=data[sex==1,])```
		```exp((modbs1$coefficients[2]))```
		```exp(confint(modbs1))```
		```modbs2=glm(cbind(hivpos,hivneg) ~idu,```
		``` family=binomial,```
		```data=data[sex==2,])```
		```exp((modbs2$coefficients[2]))```
		```exp(confint(modbs2))```
		```total1=total[sex==1]```

Question	Program	Codes
| | | ```
modps1=glm(hivpos~idu,family=poisson, offset=log
  (total1), data=data[sex==1,])
exp((modps1$coefficients[2]))
exp(confint(modps1))
total2=total[sex==2]
modps2=glm(hivpos~idu,family=poisson, offset=log
  (total2), data=data[sex==2,])
exp((modps2$coefficients[2]))
exp(confint(modps2))
``` |
| | SPSS | ```
**Logistic regression

TEMPORARY.
SELECT IF (sex=1).
GENLIN hivpos OF total BY idu (ORDER=DESCENDING)
/MODEL idu
DISTRIBUTION=binomial LINK=LOGIT
/PRINT MODELINFO SOLUTION(EXPONENTIATED).

TEMPORARY.
SELECT IF (sex=2).
GENLIN hivpos OF total BY idu (ORDER=DESCENDING)
/MODEL idu
DISTRIBUTION=binomial LINK=LOGIT
/PRINT MODELINFO SOLUTION(EXPONENTIATED).

** Poisson model

TEMPORARY.
SELECT IF (sex=1).
GENLIN hivpos BY idu (ORDER=DESCENDING)
/MODEL idu OFFSET=ltotal
DISTRIBUTION=POISSON LINK=LOG
/PRINT MODELINFO SOLUTION(EXPONENTIATED).
TEMPORARY.
SELECT IF (sex=2).
GENLIN hivpos BY idu (ORDER=DESCENDING)
/MODEL idu OFFSET=ltotal
DISTRIBUTION=POISSON LINK=LOG
/PRINT MODELINFO SOLUTION(EXPONENTIATED).
``` |
| (c) | STATA | ```
quietly xi: glm hivpos i.idu*i.sex,fam(bin total)
estimate store model1
quietly xi: glm hivpos i.idu i.sex,fam(bin total)
lrtest model1 .
quietly xi: glm hivpos i.idu*i.sex,fam(poi) lnoff
  (total)
estimate store model1
``` |
```

Question	Program	Codes
		`quietly xi: glm hivpos i.idu i.sex, fam(poi) lnoff`
		`  (total)`
		`lrtest model1 .`
	SAS	`proc logistic descending;`
		`class idu (ref='0');`
		`model hivpos/total=idu|sex;`
		`contrast 'interaction' idu*sex 1;`
		`proc genmod;`
		`class idu (ref='0') sex (ref='1')/param=effect;`
		`model hivpos/total=idu|sex/link=log dist=poi;`
		`contrast 'interaction' idu*sex 1 -1;`
		`run;`
	R	`modbc=glm(cbind(hivpos,hivneg)~idu + sex,`
		`  family=binomial,data=data)`
		`modbi=glm(cbind(hivpos,hivneg)~idu*sex,`
		`  family=binomial,`
		`data=data)`
		`anova(modbc, modbi,test="LRT")`
		`modpc=glm(hivpos~idu+sex,family=poisson, offset=log`
		`  (total), data=data)`
		`modpi=glm(hivpos~idu*sex,family=poisson, offset=log`
		`  (total), data=data)`
		`anova(modpc, modpi,test="LRT")`
	SPSS	`** Logistic regression`
		`GENLIN hivpos OF total BY idu sex (ORDER=DESCENDING)`
		`/MODEL idu sex idu*sex`
		`DISTRIBUTION=binomial LINK=LOGIT`
		`/PRINT MODELINFO SOLUTION(EXPONENTIATED).`
		`** Poisson model`
		`GENLIN hivpos BY idu sex(ORDER=DESCENDING)`
		`/MODEL idu sex idu*sex OFFSET=ltotal`
		`DISTRIBUTION=POISSON LINK=LOG`
		`/PRINT MODELINFO SOLUTION(EXPONENTIATED).`

Index

Applications of Regression Models in Epidemiology, First Edition. Erick Suárez,
Cynthia M. Pérez, Roberto Rivera, and Melissa N. Martínez.
© 2017 John Wiley & Sons, Inc. Published 2017 by John Wiley & Sons, Inc.